Encyclopedia of Chinese and U.S. Patent Herbal Medicines

Encyclopedia of Chinese and U.S. Patent Herbal Medicines

Chongyun Liu, O.M.D., L.Ac.
Yong Deng, O.M.D.
with Andrew McIntyre, L.Ac.

KEATS PUBLISHING
LOS ANGELES
NTC/Contemporary Publishing Group

Encyclopedia of Chinese and U.S. Patent Herbal Medicines is intended solely for educational and informational purposes and not as medical advice. Please consult with a medical or health professional if you have any questions about your health.

Library of Congress Cataloging-in-Publication Data

Liu, Chongyun.
Encyclopedia of Chinese and U.S. patent herbal medicines / Chongyun Liu, Young Deng, with Andrew McIntyre.
p. cm.
Includes index.
ISBN 0-87983-891-4 (pbk.)
1. Herbs—Therapeutic use Encyclopedias. 2. Materia medica, Vegetable—China Encyclopedias. 3. Materia medica, Vegetable—United States Encyclopedias. 4. Medicine, Chinese Encyclopedias. I. Deng, Yong. II. McIntyre, Andrew. III. Title.
RM666.H33L56 1999
615'.321'03—dc21 99-26881
CIP

Interior design by Cheryl Carrington

Published by Keats Publishing
A division of NTC/Contemporary Publishing Group, Inc.
4255 West Touhy Avenue, Lincolnwood, Illinois 60646-1975 U.S.A.

Printed in the United States of America

International Standard Book Number: 0-87983-891-4

10 9 8 7 6 5 4 3 2 1

Contents

Foreword

Chinese prepared medicines, popularly referred to as "patent medicines," are for the most part no longer secret; they are family and medical formulas passed down over generations. This book uses the term *patent medicine* to maintain the popular terminology. These over-the-counter preparations represent hundreds of classical Chinese formulas proven empirically over hundreds of years. Many different forms of patent medicines are used depending on their applications—from huge pills neatly packed in wax and plastic to preserve freshness to modern pharmaceutical-style preparations. It is useful to note that the term *herb* is translated from the Chinese with a very general definition; in China, herbs include animals, flora, and minerals.

The American image of the local corner pharmacy takes on an entirely different appearance in China when one walks into a famous herbal pharmacy, such as the Tong Ren Tang Pharmacy in Beijing. Operated by the same family for more than 317 years, it has dispensed patent medicines to generations of Chinese and for many years catered exclusively to Chinese royalty. With an impeccable reputation, this pharmacy and the factory that produces its medicines have set the pace in China for what is now a global export business. Many of China's neighbors produce and export patent medicines as well, often based on well-known traditional Chinese formulas.

Although China itself seems to have established a fair level of control over herbal medicine manufacturing, dispensing, and export, there are growing concerns in the West about quality control and safe manufacturing standards. In particular, there is great concern over the use of endangered animal species, adulterants, toxic contaminants, and pesticides in China and other Asian countries. Despite the level of respect many practitioners have for some herbal medicine factories in China, this is a growing concern. Many Chinese companies now originate in America, and follow higher quality control standards and show more sensitivity regarding these issues.Versions of most of the traditional Chinese patent formulas are now produced in and marketed out of America. Additionally, these American companies have developed some unique and effective variations on the ancient patent medicines. It is interesting to note that the growing trend in America toward improved manufacturing practices and herb standardization are beginning to be exported to China.

Dr. Liu and Dr. Deng have written a superb clinical therapeutic guide for the use of patent medicines. Their book should be viewed as a resource to help practitioners make the transition from the use of Chinese-manufactured formulas to those produced in America for the reasons cited above. This book presents an approach to patent medicine published here for the first time. This information is essential to all practitioners using any Chinese patent formulas. The reader will find Chinese patent medicines described along with the American ones to aid in this transition. This book is a valuable addition to the literature on Chinese medicine and will contribute to providing safe, effective, affordable, and environmentally sensitive medicines to humankind.

— MARK NOLTING, N.D., L.AC.

Acknowledgments

As is the case in any endeavor, the behind-the-scenes help of many individuals made this book possible. The authors would like to thank Ian Bier, N.D., L.Ac.; Greg Dember, L.Ac.; Susan Matsuo, R.Ph.; and Xiaosong Wang, M.D. (China), L.Ac., for their invaluable suggestions, assistance, and support.

For their extensive technical aid and many late nights of hard work, the authors extend their grateful thanks to Prassert Ngamsiripol, M.D. (China), L.Ac., and Jonathan Chang, M.D., L.Ac.

And finally, many thanks to Andrew McIntyre, L.Ac., for his conceptual and textual editing of this book.

Introduction

Background of Patent Herbal Medicines

Chinese prepared, or "patent," herbal medicines have their roots in an herbal tradition that stretches back more than five thousand years. What began in ancient times as courageous, if not foolhardy, trial-and-error experimentation with individual herbs eventually grew into a coherent classification system. Herbs were classified according to their properties and what they treated. Discoveries about multiple-herb formulas arose when practitioners recognized that by targeting different aspects of an illness, combinations of herbs could treat illnesses more effectively than could single herbs. Herbalists found, for example, that in a common cold formula, one herb might address fever, while another could treat sweating. Another herb in the formula might harmonize the activity of all the others, creating a synergy that enhanced their efficiency.

As practitioners shared information and knowledge increased, many of these formulas became established in Traditional Chinese Medicine (TCM). They are now referred to as "classical" formulas because of their effectiveness and their origins in antiquity.

They are still used. When writing a custom formula for a patient, herbalists usually begin with a core, classical formula and then build on and customize that formula to meet the specific needs of the case. Many of these classical formulas became the basis for what we now call Chinese patent medicines.

Originally created by families or specific healing traditions, patent medicines were formulas whose exact ingredients and amounts were kept secret. To maintain this secrecy, the medicines were prepared in advance, instead of being mixed or prepared as needed. The herbs were typically ground up and fashioned into a pill-like form, or were dispensed as a powdered mixture. Plasters, or compresses, were another common form for patent medicines.

Because they were convenient and economical in addition to being effective, Chinese patent medicines became popular and are now the most common way Chinese medicinal herbs are taken. These days, with few exceptions, the ingredients and their amounts are known and have become standardized. Patent medicines from China now typically are dispensed as small black spherical pills of ground herbs, packaged in amber bottles listing the name and ingredients on the label; compresses are still popular, as well.

Although patent medicines were available in the United States prior to former President Richard Nixon's trip to China in 1972, this was when Chinese herbal and patent medicines were first introduced to the U.S. population at large. Almost all the patent medicines available in this country at that time were imported from China. Demand for and interest in Chinese medicine in the United States grew gradually for the first ten to fifteen years after 1972, but have grown significantly in the last ten years.

The increase in Chinese medicine in the United States has highlighted two significant problems with Chinese-produced patent medicines. The first has persisted throughout the history of patent medicines: quality control. Production methods for patent formulas have been unscientific and have not adhered to stringent guidelines. Dosages for ingredients can be inaccurate. Less costly alternatives are sometimes substituted for standard ingredients without changing container labels to inform the consumer. Occasionally, the entire manufacturing process is altered, resulting in a different form or size of the herbal mix, but the packaging stays the same and does not indicate dosage changes or variants in intake instructions.

Another problem concerns the ingredients themselves. Pesticide use in cultivating herbs in China is widespread, leading to high levels of pesticide residues in the final product. Sulfites are employed in the production of most patent medicines made in China. Significant levels of heavy metals have been found in Chinese patent medicines. And many patent formulas call for the use of animal parts from animals now on the endangered species list. Indeed, the demand created by their use in herbal medicines continues to be one of the primary forces driving these animals to the brink of extinction. Although a law preventing the use of endangered species in herbal medicines was passed in China in 1996, use of these animals persists.

These problems are in the process of being resolved. The first U.S. manufacturers arrived on the scene in the 1970s. (Jade Pharmacy, for example, was founded in 1971.) Consumer demand and U.S. legal requirements led to a marked increase in quality control with greatly improved and much safer production methods. The strict labeling requirements of the U.S. Food and Drug Administration (FDA), along with the Fish and Wildlife Service's governance over endangered species, provided the legal impetus for these improvements. The new U.S. companies removed or found effective substitutes for controversial animal ingredients and avoided the use of sprayed or otherwise contaminated herbs. In the midst of resolving these difficulties, however, a practical problem has arisen with the arrival of the U.S. companies.

Practitioners of Chinese herbal medicine usually learn patent formulas by their Chinese names. U.S. companies, however, frequently give their products (often identical to their Chinese counterparts) English names. Jade Pharmacy, for instance, has combined the two patent formulas *Yin Qiao* and *Sang Chu Yin* to create their *Prime Response*. The patent medicine *Xiao Yao Wan* is now Golden Flower's *Bupleurum* and *Tang Kuei Formula*. Often, the English name used by U.S. companies is the translation of the patent medicine's Chinese name. Often, however, it is not. And many practitioners do not know the English meanings of Chinese names anyway. This has created some confusion. While it is entirely possible for practitioners to figure out which American formula corresponds to which Chinese patent medicine, the process can be time consuming, especially when different U.S. companies call the same Chinese patent equivalent by different names.

At the moment, there is no comprehensive guide to sort through this situation. Due to the high quality of U.S. herbal products and the assurance that they use no endangered animals, demand for U.S.-made patent medicines is growing rapidly. One of the purposes of this book, therefore, is to aid students and practitioners in figuring out which U.S. product corresponds to which Chinese patent medicine, and how U.S. products correspond to each other.

At the same time, it is helpful to have the conditions being treated presented along with the patent medicines used to treat them. This is a useful refresher for those familiar with TCM, but is especially beneficial for health care practitioners not trained in TCM who wish to use Chinese patent formulas. A brief description of the disease in Western and TCM terms, along with etiology, pathogenesis, and treatment, are presented. For further information on the information in this book and how to use it, please see the following section, How to Use This Book.

Fifty-five conditions have been included. While the scope of this book is not intended to be all-encompassing, the conditions included represent much of what an acupuncturist or herbalist will see in his or her clinical practice. Also, many conditions not given their own section headings are covered, although under different names. Rheumatoid arthritis, for example, will be found under the section for Bi Syndrome, while cough can be found in the sections on Common Cold and Asthma. Please check the Symptom Reference Index for conditions not given their own sections.

About the U.S. Companies Included in This Book

There are currently many companies producing versions of Chinese patent medicines in the United States. New companies are started each year while others have ceased operations. Some are small and offer a few specialized products, while others have larger product offerings and are more comprehensive in scope. Due to logistical constraints and concern for longstanding reputation, the latter companies were selected for inclusion in this book. These are the larger, better-known companies that have existed the longest among the manufacturers. The authors would like to mention here that exclusion from this book is not meant in any way to confer or suggest that a company's products are substandard. The authors take full responsibility for the companies selected. As more U.S. companies become established, they will likely be included in later revised editions of this book.

Please refer to the following list for the names of the U.S. companies and their abbreviations, as used throughout this book.

Company Abbreviations

Chinese Herb Company	CHC
Chinese Modular Solutions	CMS
East Tao Herb Pharmacy	ETHP
Golden Flower Chinese Herbs	GFCH
Health Concerns	HC
Jade Pharmacy	Jade
K'an Herbals	K'an
Long Life Herb Pharmacy	LLHP
Metagenics	MG
Pacific BioLogic	PB
ProBotanixx	Pro
The Three Treasures	TTT
Women's Treasure Formulae	WT

How to Use This Book

This book has been designed for easy accessibility. It is intended to serve as a frequently used, reader-friendly guide for acupuncturists, herbalists, and other health care practitioners. It should be easy for health care providers wishing to use Chinese herbal remedies or their U.S. equivalents to find the necessary information to do so. To aid those unfamiliar with TCM, U.S. patent medicines useful for treating each subtype of a condition have been included for each condition.

PART I: Diseases and Conditions

The first part of this book contains basic syndromes and diseases an acupuncturist or Chinese herbalist is likely to encounter. It contains most of the conditions acupuncture students learn about in their therapeutics courses. The diseases and conditions are presented alphabetically. A brief description is provided for each, usually in terms of both Western medicine and TCM, followed by its etiology and pathology according to TCM. A table is then provided, also in the context of TCM, for each that includes its subtype, manifestations, treatment principle, the classical formulas and Chinese patent medicines recommended, and U.S. equivalents of the Chinese formulas. It should be noted here that the term *equivalents* is used somewhat loosely, as there will occasionally be differences from the exact ingredients of the Chinese formulas. The U.S. equivalents often do match up exactly with their Chinese counterparts, but those that do not, yet are similar enough to treat the same conditions, are called *equivalents*.

A table format is employed to facilitate efficiency when using this book. This book is intended for use in the clinical setting, where time considerations are important. Having the subtypes, symptoms, treatment principles, and corresponding patent medicines all in the same section will greatly improve speed and accuracy in the clinical setting. Comparisons among subtypes can be performed quickly for accurate diagnoses with this format.

The reader may also notice that occasionally no Chinese patent medicines are listed for a given subtype of a condition. In these instances, it is usually because the classical formula itself, as opposed to a patent medicine, is used in a dried herb-based decoction or powdered form. The U.S. products listed in these cases are derived directly from the classical formulas.

It should also be mentioned that due to the paradigm of Chinese medicine in which outward manifestations are believed to reveal inner conditions, there may appear to those unfamiliar with TCM to be unusual overlaps and redundancies. Examples of this are headache and sore throat. Each is a common, secondary symptom of other conditions and will be found in several sections, such as Hypertension or Common Cold, yet each receives its own section as a primary condition viewed in isolation. While there are similarities to Western medicine in this regard, the reader will find that this situation applies more frequently in TCM, where what might be considered symptoms in Western medicine are viewed as conditions in themselves. Where necessary, the distinction is made and should be easy to follow. Many of the conditions presented, however, do follow Western-style classification, though the diagnosis and treatment is presented according to TCM.

PART II: Cross-Reference of Chinese and U.S. Patent Herbal Medicines

The second part of this book is for practitioners who already know the herbal formula they wish to use or for those who want quick comparisons of the same formula among the various U.S. companies. The traditional Chinese formulas are listed alphabetically according to their Pinyin name in one column with their U.S. equivalents in another column. Many of the practitioners who use this book will already know the TCM diagnosis and traditional herbal formula they want but may not know all the U.S. counterparts. This section is intended to serve as a quick reference for such practitioners.

PART III: U.S. Formula Ingredients List

The third part of this book contains more detailed information about the U.S. formulas. This is for practitioners who want to know the individual ingredients of the U.S. formulas presented in the previous two parts and provides information regarding possible contraindications and other relevant notes.

PART I

Diseases and Conditions

Abdominal Pain

Abdominal pain is a common symptom characterized by pain in the area below the epigastrium and above the suprapubic hair margin. The abdominal pain discussed here does not include that caused by an acute abdominal condition that requires emergency surgical intervention.

Etiology and pathology

1. Accumulation of cold in the interior
2. Milk and food stagnation
3. Deficient cold of the middle jiao
4. Qi and blood stagnation

Differentiation and treatment

U.S. formulas that can be used in all types include *Yellow Xiao Yao San* (ETHP) and *GI-335* (Pro).

Type	Manifestations	Treatment Principle	Chinese Formula	U.S. Formula and Manufacturer
Accumulation of cold in the abdomen	Sudden onset of abdominal pain that can be relieved by warmth and aggravated by cold, pale complexion, dark purple lips, cold limbs, vomiting, diarrhea, profuse clear urine; white and slippery tongue coating	Disperse cold	Classical Formulas: 1. *Yang Zang San* 2. *Da Huang Fu Zi Tang*	1. *Purge Cold* (CMS)
Milk and food retention	Distending abdominal pain aggravated by pressure, foul belching, sour regurgitation, flatulence, diarrhea with foul-smelling stool, pain relieved after passing stool; thick and greasy tongue coating	Promote digestion and remove food stagnation	Classical Formulas: 1. *Xiang Sha Ping Wei San* Patent Medicines 1. *Bao He Wan*	1. *Meal Mover* (CMS) 2. *Purge Qi* (CMS) 3. *Morning Glory (ETHP)*

Type	Manifestations	Treatment Principle	Chinese Formula	U.S. Formula & Manufacturer
Middle jiao deficient cold	Intermittent, lingering dull pain in the abdomen with desire for warmth and pressure, pale complexion, fatigue, cold limbs, poor appetite, abdominal distention after meals, loose stool; pale tongue with white coating	Warm the middle jiao and tonify deficiency	Classical Formulas: 1. *Xiao Jian Zhong Tang* + *Li Zhong Tang* Patent Medicines: 1. *Fu Zi Li Zhong Wan*	1. *Purge Cold* (CMS) 2. *Astragalus Formula* (GFCH)
Qi and blood stagnation	Distending or sharp abdominal pain, aggravated by pressure or masses in the abdomen, dark lips; dark purple tongue body	Circulate qi and blood and relieve the obstruction	Classical Formulas: 1. *Shao Fu Zhu Yu Tang* Patent Medicines: 1. *Yan Hu Zhi Tong Pian*	1. *Corydalis Formula* (GFCH) 2. *Purge Blood* (CMS) 3. *Invigorate the Collaterals* (K'an) 4. *San Qi Tablets* (GFCH)

Acne

Acne is a skin condition consisting of papules, blackheads or whiteheads, pustules, inflamed nodules, and cysts that usually appear on the face, upper chest, shoulders, and upper back. TCM groups the subcategories of acne into one group, though it does place emphasis on *acne vulgaris*, or adolescent acne. Thus, TCM calls acne "adolescent blemish."

Etiology and pathology

There are generally two types of acne.

1. Oil acne, caused mainly by damp heat of the stomach and spleen, in which damp heat accumulates and steams out distributing in the skin
2. Adolescent acne, or climacteric acne, caused mainly by a disharmony in the Chong and Ren meridians (corresponding to hormonal imbalance) in which the skin pores fail to open and close properly

Differentiation and treatment

Treatment is directed toward eliminating heat toxins, cleansing the lungs, and harmonizing the Chong and Ren meridians. Certain lifestyle behaviors are considered important in the treatment of acne. Dietary adjustments include the avoidance of high-fat foods, spicy foods, alcohol, and coffee. Smoking is also to be avoided, as are stress, constipation, and wearing makeup. U.S. formulas that can be used in all types include *Q.B.R.* (ETHP) and *SK-741* (Pro).

Type	Manifestations	Treatment Principle	Chinese Formula	U.S. Formula and Manufacturer
Stomach and spleen damp heat	Skin eruptions on face, back, and chest, oily and uncomfortable skin sensations, pimples or lesions with pus or blackheads, oozing lesions, possible constipation and halitosis; red tongue body with yellow greasy coating, rapid slippery pulse	Eliminate heat toxins, transform and eliminate damp	Classical Formulas: 1. *Yin Chen Hao Tang + Pi Pa Qing Fei Yin* 2. *Pu Ji Xiao Du Yin + Da Chai Hu Tang* Patent Medicines: 1. *Huang Lian Shang Qing Pian*	1. *Skin Balance + Coptis Purge Fire* (HC) 2. *CoptiDetox* (K'an) 3. *Coptis Relieve Toxicity Formula* (GFCH) 4. *Detox Compound* (CHC) 5. *Purge Heat + Phlogisticlean* (CMS) 6. *LD-477* (Pro) 7. *Liver Detox* (Jade) 8. *Flavor 21* (ETHP)
Disharmony between the Chong and Ren	Acne that comes and goes with menstrual period, may be accompanied by irregular menstruation or dysmenorrhea; dark red or purple tongue with thin yellow coating, wiry or thready, rapid pulse	Harmonize Chong and Ren, soothe liver qi	Classical Formulas: 1. *Dan Zhi Xiao Yao San* 2. *Er Xian Tang* Patent Medicines: 1. *Yi Mu Tiao Jing Wan*	1. *Smooth Passage + Break Into a Smile* (TTT) 2. *Woman's Balance + Two Immortals* (HC) 3. *Heavenly Water* (HC) — heart and spleen deficiency 4. *Jade Shining + Er Xian Tang Plus* (ETHP) 5. *Women's Journey* (Jade and K'an) 6. *Wise Woman's Well* (CMS) 7. *PM-637 + ME-523* (Pro) 8. *Free and Easy Wanderer Plus* (GFCH)

Amenorrhea

Amenorrhea refers to the condition among women aged eighteen or older who have never menstruated or women who have not menstruated for more than three months after a normal menstrual cycle has previously been established. Absence of menses during pregnancy or breast-feeding is a normal physiological phenomenon. Amenorrhea due to congenital maldevelopment and defect is not considered here.

Etiology and Pathology

1. Liver and kidney deficiency
2. Qi and blood deficiency
3. Qi and blood stagnation
4. Obstruction of phlegm damp

Differentiation and treatment

U.S. formulas that can be used in all types include *Astra Essence* (HC).

Type	Manifestations	Treatment Principle	Chinese Formula	U.S. Formula & Manufacturer
Liver and kidney deficiency	No menses over the age of eighteen, or delayed or scanty menstrual flow gradually developing to ammenorrhea, weak constitution, dizziness, tinnitus, soreness and weakness in the lumbar region and knees; pale tongue body, scanty coating, deep and weak pulse	Tonify and nourish the liver and kidney	Classical Formulas: 1. *Zuo Gui Wan + You Gui Wan* Patent Medicines: 1. *Gui Shen Wan* 2. *Zuo Gui Wan + You Gui Wan* 3. *Gui Ling Ji*	1. *Unicorn Pearl* (WT) Yin Xu 2. *Ease Journey-Yin* (WT) 3. *Quiet Contemplative* (Jade and K'an) Yang xu 4. *Ease Journey-Yang* (WT) 5. *Warm the Mansion* (WT)

Type	Manifestations	Treatment Principle	Chinese Formula	U.S. Formula and Manufacturer
Qi and blood deficiency	Delayed and scanty menstrual flow gradually developing to ammenorrhea, lassitude, dizziness, palpitations, shortness of breath, poor appetite, sallow complexion; pale tongue body, white coating, thready and weak pulse	Tonify qi and blood	Classical Formulas: 1. *Ren Shen Yang Rong Tang* 2. *Ba Zhen Tang* 3. *Gui Pi Tang* Patent Medicines: 1. *Ren Shen Yang Rong Wan* 2. *Gui Pi Wan* 3. *Ba Zhen Yi Mu Wan*	1. *Precious Sea* (WT) 2. *Women's Precious* (K'an and Jade) 3. *Eight Treasures* (HC) 4. *Gather Vitality* (K'an and Jade)
Qi and blood stagnation	Ammenorrhea, mental depression or irritability, distention and fullness in the chest and hypochondrium, lower abdominal pain aggravated by pressure, dark purple complexion; dark purple tongue body or purple spots on the tongue, deep wiry or deep uneven pulse	Circulate qi and blood, regulate menstruation	Classical Formulas: 1. *Xue Fu Zhu Yu Tang*	1. *Women's Rhythm* (K'an and Jade) 2. *Women's Chamber* (K'an) 3. *Women's Palace* (Jade)
Phlegm damp retention	Prolonged menstrual cycle with scanty flow gradually developing to ammenorrhea, obesity, distress in the chest and epigastrium, nausea, profuse sputum, poor appetite, lassitude, profuse, sticky, and white vaginal discharge; white sticky tongue coating, slippery pulse	Resolve phlegm and restore normal menstruation	Classical Formulas: 1. *Cang Fu Dao Tan Wan* + *Fu Shou San* Patent Medicines: 1. *Cang Fu Dao Tan Wan*	1. *Clear the Palace* (WT) 2. *Lucid Channel and Lucid Clarity* (K'an and Jade) 3. *Disperse the Moisture* (CMS)

Aphthae (Canker Sores)

Apthae is a disease of the mouth, characterized by ulcerative lesions on the oral mucosa, both sides of the tongue, the palate, or the gums. Although it occurs in all age groups, it is most common in children, particularly infants. In Western medicine, it is called ulcerative stomatitis or aphthous stomatitis, and is known commonly as canker sores.

Etiology and pathology

1. Excessive intake of fat, sweet, rich, and warm food leading to heat
2. Yin xu constitution, febrile diseases causing deficient heat

Differentiation and treatment

U.S. formulas that can be used in all types include *Mountain Sophora* (ETHP).

Type	Manifestations	Treatment Principle	Chinese Formula	U.S. Formula and Manufacturer
Excessive heat accumulation	Ulcers or erosion in the oral mucosa, refusal of food due to pain, irritability, halitosis, salivation, dark urine, constipation, fever, flushed face; red tongue body with yellow coating	Clear heat, purge fire and detoxify	Classical Formulas: 1. *Lian Ge San* 2. *Qing Wei San* 3. *Gan Lu Xiao Du Dan* 4. *Dao Chi San* Patent Medicines: 1. *Niu Huang Jie Du Pian* 2. *Niu Huang Shang Qing Wan* 3. *Tao Chih Pian*	1. *Coptis Relieve Toxicity Formula* (GFCH) 2. *CoptiDetox* (K'an) 3. *Five Detox* (LLHP)
Deficient fire flaring up	Few or scattered ulcers over the oral mucosa with light color, slight pain, flushed cheeks, feverish sensation in the palms and soles, dry mouth with no desire for drinking; red tongue with little or no coating	Tonify yin and clear deficient fire	Classical Formulas: 1. *Zhi Bai Di Huang Wan* Patent Medicines: 1. *Zhi Bai Di Huang Wan*	1. *Temper Fire* (K'an and Jade) 2. *Rehmannia and Scrophularia Formula* (GFCH) 3. *Nine Flavor Tea* (HC)

Asthma

Asthma is a condition characterized mainly by prolonged attacks of dyspnea (labored breathing) with wheezing, prolonged exhalation, and difficulty lying down during an attack. TCM divides asthma into two main types: "sounding" asthma and "soundless" asthma. The former is marked by dyspnea with wheezing, the latter by hasty, shallow breathing with opening of the mouth and occasional raising of the shoulders to aid breathing. Because, in TCM, these two types are not markedly different in their etiology and pathogenesis and may appear simultaneously, the two are treated as one illness. Asthma may occur in any of the four seasons, though more so in the colder months. It includes the diagnoses of bronchial asthma and asthmatic bronchitis in Western medicine.

Etiology and pathology

1. Wind cold invades the lung, impairing the lung's function of dispersing the qi
2. Improper diet impairs the spleen's ability in transforming and transporting, leading to the accumulation of dampness which in turn produces phlegm; prolonged accumulation of phlegm may turn into heat that can cause the obstruction of qi
3. Prolonged illness and protracted cough leads to impairment of lung qi
4. Overstrain or excessive sexual activity damages kidney essence and depletes kidney qi, resulting in the inability of the kidney to receive qi

Differentiation and treatment

U.S. formulas that can be used in all types include *Clear Air* (HC) and *Clear Qi* (TTT).

Type	Manifestations	Treatment Principle	Chinese Formula	U.S. Formula and Manufacturer
Dormant cold in the lung—acute stage	DifficultY respiration, cough with shortness of breath and wheezing sounds, thin clear or white sputum, cold limbs, grAy facial complexion; white or white greasy tongue coating, superficial tense or superficial slippery pulse	Dispel pathogenic cold from the lung, eliminate phlegm, and relieve asthma	Classical Formulas: 1. *Ma Huang Tang* 2. *Xiao Qing Long Tang* Patent Medicines: 1. *Gan Mao Ling* 2. *Sang Ju Pian* 3. *Xiao Ke Chai Syrup*	1. *Minor Blue Dragon* (HC) 2. *AS-135* (Pro) 3. *Minor Bluegreen Dragon Formula* (GFCH) *Note:* If external cold signs present, add *Prime Rescue* (Jade) or *CO-195 (Pro)*

Type	Manifestations	Treatment Principle	Chinese Formula	U.S. Formula and Manufacturer
Phlegm heat in the lung—acute stage	Quick, shallow breathing with high-pitched wheezing, fever, flushed face, thick yellow sputum that is difficult to expectorate, congested feeling in the chest and epigastric region, thirst with desire for cold drinks, yellow urine, constipation; yellow, greasy tongue coating, rapid, slippery pulse	Clear phlegm heat, circulate lung qi, and stop asthma	Classical Formulas: 1. *Ding Chuan Tang* 2. *Ma Xing Shi Gan Tang* 3. *Zhi Sou Ding Chuan Wan* Patent Medicines: 1. *Qi Guan Yan Wan* 2. *Qi Guan Yan Ke Shou Tan Chai Wan*	1. *AS-137* (Pro) 2. *Clear Air* (HC) 3. *Chest Relief* (CMS) *Note*: With profuse yellow sputum, add *Fritellaria and Pinnellia Syrup* (GFCH).
Spleen and lung qi deficiency—remission stage	Reluctance to speak, shortness of breath, weak cough, sweating from exertion of coughing, pale complexion, poor appetite, edema in face and limbs; pale tongue body with white coating, soft, weak pulse	Strengthen spleen and lung qi	Classical Formulas: 1. *Liu Jun Zi Tang + Yu Ping Feng San* Patent Medicines: 1. *Li Fei* 2. *Xiang Sha Liu Jun Zi Wan*	1. *Astra C* (HC) 2. *IM-401* (Pro) 3. *Prosperous Farmer* (Jade and K'an) 4. *Six Gentlemen Formula* (GFCH) 5. *Strengthen Lung* (CMS)
Lung and kidney qi deficiency—remission stage	Cough and shortness of breath aggravated by exertion of opening mouth and raising shoulders, lassitude, weakness, and soreness of lumbar region and knees, vertigo with tinnitus, nocturnal emmision, cold limbs, darkened complexion; pale tongue body, deep, thready pulse	Tonify lung and kidney qi and stop asthma	Classical Formulas: 1. *Jin Gui Shen Qi Wan* 2. *Qi Wei Du Qi Wan* 3. *Ren Shen Ge Jie San* Patent Medicines: 1. *Jin Gui Shen Qi Wan* 2. *Ge Jie Da Bu Wan*	1. *Ginseng and Gecko Herbal Formula* (HC) 2. *Dynamic Warrior* (Jade and K'an) 3. *Strengthen Kidney* (CMS) 4. *Mo Plus* (ETHP)

Beng Lou (Uterine Bleeding)

Beng Lou is a TCM term that denotes irregular vaginal hemorrhage and corresponds to functional uterine bleeding in Western medicine. Beng (metrorrhagia) is massive uterine bleeding characterized by sudden onset and profuse quantity, while Lou (metrostaxis) is chronic, mild, scanty bleeding marked by incessant dripping of blood from the uterus outside the normal menstrual cycle. Although one condition is acute and the other is chronic, Beng and Lou share similarities in etiology. As this disease develops, the two often transform into each other. Massive bleeding (Beng) may deplete the qi and blood, consequently transforming into Lou. Likewise, if Lou is not treated, it may eventually develop into Beng.

Etiology and pathology

Deficiency Type

1. Spleen qi deficiency
2. Kidney deficiency

Excess Type

1. Blood heat
2. Lower jiao damp heat
3. Blood stagnation

Differentiation and treatment

U.S. formulas that can be used in all types include *Hemmorease* (K'an) and *Restrain the Flow* (WT).

Type	Manifestations	Treatment Principle	Chinese Formula	U.S. Formula and Manufacturer
Spleen qi deficiency	Uterine bleeding marked by light red and thin blood, pale complexion, fatigue, shortness of breath, reluctance to speak, poor appetite; pale tongue body, thin white coating, thready and weak pulse	Invigorate qi, tonify the middle jiao, and stop bleeding	Classical Formulas: 1. *Gu Ben Zhi Beng Tang* 2. *Gui Pi Tang* Patent Medicines: 1. *Gui Pi Wan*	1. *Restrain the Flow* (WT) 2. *Gather Vitality* (K'an and Jade) 3. *Energy A* (ETHP)
Kidney yang deficiency	Light red and thin blood, lower abdominal cold pain, intolerance of coldness, cold extremities, loose stool; pale tongue body, white coating, deep thin pulse	Warm and tonify kidney yang and consolidate the menses	Classical Formulas: KIDNEY YANG XU 1. *You Gui Wan + Rou gui, Dang gui, Huang qi, Fu pen zi, Chi shi zhi* Patent Medicines: KIDNEY YANG XU 1. *You Gui Wan* 2. *Ting Gui Shen Qi Wan*	1. *Ease the Journey–Yang* (WT) 2. *Planting Seeds* (WT) 3. *Energy D* (ETHP)

Type	Manifestations	Treatment Principle	Chinese Formula	U.S. Formula and Manufacturer
Kidney yin deficiency	Scanty bleeding with bright red blood, dizziness, tinnitus, five center fever, insomnia, night sweats, soreness and weakness of the low back and knees; red tongue body, scanty coating, thin and rapid pulse	Nourish kidney yin, clear deficient fire, and stop bleeding	Classical Formulas: 1. *Zuo Gui Wan* + *Er Zhi Wan* 2. *Zhi Bai Di Huang Wan*	1. *Nourish Yin and Restrain the Flow* (WT) 2. *Temper Fire* (K'an and Jade) 3. *Rehmannia and Scrophularia Formula* (GFCH) *Note:* Use any of the above in combination with *Clear Empty-Heat* and *Cool the Menses* (WT) to increase the action of cooling blood.
Blood heat	Sudden onset of profuse or prolonged continuous vaginal bleeding, deep red in color and thick in quality, restlessness, irritability, thirst; red or dark red tongue body, yellow or thick yellow coating, slippery, rapid pulse	Clear heat, cool blood, and stop bleeding	Classical Formulas: 1. *Qing Re Gu Jing Tang* Patent Medicines: 1. *Gu Jing Wan*	1. *Cool the Menses* (WT) *Note:* For presence of liver fire, combine with *Free and Easy Wanderer Plus* (GFCH).
Damp heat	Uterine bleeding with foul-smelling yellow green leukorrhea, itching and pain in the vulva; red tongue body with yellow greasy coating, soft and rapid pulse	Clear heat and remove damp	Classical Formulas: 1. *Long Dan Xie Gan Tang* Patent Medicines: 1. *Long Dan Xie Gan Wan*	1. *Quell Fire* (K'an and Jade) 2. *Gentiana Drain Fire Formula* (GFCH)
Blood stasis	Dark purple blood with blood clots, abdominal pain aggravated by pressure and alleviated after passing out clots; dark purple tongue body, deep and uneven pulse	Promote blood circulation to remove the blood stasis and arrest bleeding	Classical Formulas: 1. *Si Wu Tang* + *Shi Xiao San, San Qi, Qian Cao Tang, Wu zei gu* Patent Medicines: 1. *Yun Nan Bai Yao*	1. *Invigorate Blood* and *Stem the Flow* (WT)

Benign Prostate Hypertrophy

Benign prostate hypertrophy (BHP) is enlargement of the prostate gland, a common occurrence in men over fifty years of age. BHP causes urinary difficulties such as frequent urination, dysuria, urinary tract infections, urinary incontinence, hematuria, and urinary retention. In TCM it is known as Long Bi and has a long history of successful treatment with herbs and acupuncture.

Etiology and pathology

The lower jiao, the kidney, and urinary bladder are the organs involved in BHP.

1. Damp heat accumulation in the lower jiao
2. Kidney qi/yang deficiency leads to qi hua function failure
3. Blood stagnation causes urinary blockage

Differentiation and treatment

BHP is usually differentiated into three types. Treatment is directed toward transforming damp, invigorating qi and blood and strengthening the kidney. U.S. formulas that can be used in all types include *Prostate Combination* (CHC) and *PR-681* (Pro).

Type	Manifestations	Treatment Principle	Chinese Formula	U.S. Formula and Manufacturer
Damp heat	Dripping urine with pain, urine retention, bloated lower abdomen, bitter taste in the mouth, thirst without the desire to drink; red tongue body with sticky yellow coating, especially in back of the tongue, slippery rapid pulse	Transform damp and clear heat from lower jiao	Classical Formulas: 1. *Ba Zheng San* 2. *Si Hai Shu Yu Wan* Patent Medicines: 1. *Pass Wan* 2. *Shi Lin Tong*	1. *Akebia Moist Heat + Unlocking Formula* (HC) 2. *Drain the Jade Valley* (WT) 3. *Lower Burner* (Jade) 4. *UI-821* (Pro) 5. *Unlocking the Gate* (CMS) 6. *Ling Syndrome Formula* (ETHP)

Type	Manifestations	Treatment Principle	Chinese Formula	U.S. Formula and Manufacturer
Kidney qi/ yang deficiency	Difficulty urinating, scanty or dripping urination, dysuria due to lack of force to void bladder, chalky, pale complexion, low spirit, cold limbs and low back, fear of the cold, achy and weak low back and knees; pale tongue body with white coating, deep, thready slow pulse, pronounced at *chi* level	Warm kidney yang, boost qi hua function, and promote urination	Classical Formulas: 1. *Ji Sheng Shen Qi Wan* 2. *Xiang Rong Wan + Zhu Ling Tang* 3. *You Gui Wan* Patent Medicines: 1. *Ji Sheng Shen Qi Wan* 2. *You Gui Wan*	1. *Essence Chamber + Astra Essence* (HC) 2. *Strengthen the Root* (TTT) 3. *Essential Yang Formula* (GFCH) 4. *Dynamic Warrior* (Jade and K'an) 5. *Replenish Essence* (CMS) 6. *MA-511* (Pro)
Blood stagnation	Dripping and difficult urination with sharp fixed pain in lower abdomen and perineum, threadlike urine flow off and on; deep red, purple, or purple spotted tongue body, deep choppy pulse	Transform blood stasis, dredge blocked meridians, and promote urination	Classical Formulas: 1. *Shao Fu Zhu Yu Tang* 2. *Gui Zhi Fu Ling Wan* Patent Medicines: 1. *Jie Jie Wan*	1. *Unlocking Formula + Crampbark Plus* (HC) 2. *Stir Field of Elixir* (TTT) 3. *Purge Blood* (CMS) 4. *Cinnamon and Poria Formula* (GFCH) 5. *Women's Palace* (Jade) 6. *Women's Chamber* (K'an) 7. *Kai Tong Pian* (ETHP)

Bi Syndrome (Painful Obstruction Syndrome)

Bi syndrome is a Chinese disease type involving bodily aches and pains. In Chinese, *Bi* means "obstruction." Bi syndrome manifests as aching, numbness, and heavy sensations in the limbs, joints, and muscles. Swollen joints and limited movement due to poor circulation also fall under the Bi syndrome classification, as do aches and pains from qi and blood stagnation caused by exogenous pathogenic invasions. The pain in Bi syndrome can manifest as progressive pain or pain in the form of repeated attacks. Bi syndrome includes, but is not limited to, rheumatic fever, rheumatoid arthritis, rheumatoid gout, and rheumatic myofibrositis in Western medicine.

Etiology and pathology

1. Wandering Bi—mainly from wind invasion
2. Painful Bi—mainly from cold invasion
3. Fixed Bi—mainly from dampness invasion
4. Febrile Bi—mainly from heat as a result of stagnated wind, cold, or dampness
5. Stubborn Bi—chronic Bi penetrating the meridians and collateral channels, causing qi and blood stagnation

Differentiation and treatment

Treatment is directed toward moving qi and blood. U.S. formulas that can be used in all types include *AR-125* (Pro) and *Channel Flow* (HC).

Type	Manifestations	Treatment Principle	Chinese Formula	U.S. Formula and Manufacturer
Wandering Bi	Wandering pain and soreness in the limbs, joints, and muscles, particularly in the wrists, elbows, knees, and ankles, limited movements of the joints, fever with aversion to cold; thin, greasy tongue coating, and superficial, wiry pulse	Disperse wind, cold, and damp; remove the obstruction	Classical Formulas: 1. *Fang Feng Tang* Patent Medicines: 1. *Jiu Wei Qiang Huo Wan*	1. *Chase Wind, Penetrate Bone Formula* (GFCH) 2. *AR-125* (Pro)
Painful Bi	Severe, sharp, stabbing pain in the limbs and joints, fixed pain that is alleviated by warmth and aggravated by cold, pain that is better in the day and worse at night, limited movements of the joints, cold sensations in affected area, no local redness or feverish sensations; thin white tongue coating, wiry, tense pulse	Warm the channels and relieve cold, disperse wind, and resolve dampness	Classical Formulas: 1. *Wu Tou Tang* Patent Medicines: 1. *Guan Jie Yan Wan*	1. *Juan Bi Formula* (GFCH) 2. *AR-125* (Pro) 3. *TCB2 Stephania Combination* (MG) 4. *Mobility 2* (HC)

Type	Manifestations	Treatment Principle	Chinese Formula	U.S. Formula and Manufacturer
Fixed Bi	Pain and heavy sensations in fixed areas of body limbs or joints, numbness of the muscles, aggravation of symptoms on rainy days; white, greasy tongue coating, soft, moderate pulse	Resolve dampness and dredge the collaterals; disperse wind and dispel cold	Classical Formulas: 1. *Yi Yi Ren Tang* Patent Medicines: 1. *Du Huo Ji Sheng Wan*	1. *Bi Syndrome Formula* (ETHP) 2. *Meridian Circulation* (Jade and K'an)
Febrile Bi	Painful limbs or joints with localized heat sensations with redness, pain aggravated by pressure, limited movement involving one or more joints, fever, thirst with desire for cold drinks, restlessness, aversion to heat; yellow tongue coating, slippery, rapid pulse	Clear heat and dredge the collaterals; disperse wind and resolve damp	Classical Formulas: 1. *Chai Hu Gui Zhi Tang* Patent Medicines: 1. *Vine Essence*	1. *Smilax Compound* (ETHP)
Stubborn Bi	History of repeated attacks of hot or cold Bi syndrome that have deformed affected joints, possible black spots on affected joints, severe pain, limited movement *Hot type:* numbness, redness, swelling of joints, fever, thirst, scanty urine, red tongue with yellow coating *Cold type:* cold sensations in the joints, condition worsened in cold seasons, alleviation of pain by warmth; purplish, dark tongue with purplish spots, thready, hesitant pulse	Circulate qi and blood and remove obstruction	Classical Formulas: 1. *Shen Tong Zhu Yu Tang* Patent Medicines: 1. *Xiao Huo Luo Dan*	1. *Meridian Passage* (K'an and Jade) 2. *PA-623* (Pro) *Note:* For patients with weak constitution or prolonged Bi with liver and kidney deficiency, add any of the following: *Du Huo and Loranthus Formula* (GFCH), *Mobility 3* (HC), or *AR-127* (Pro).

Candidiasis

Candidiasis is infection by a yeastlike fungi, usually *Candida albicans*. While *C. albicans* forms a normal part of the flora of the gastrointestinal tract, mouth, skin, and vagina, it can cause infections in each of these areas as well as in the respiratory tract. It is thought that widespread long-term use of antibiotics may be implicated in the increased incidence of candidiasis. In TCM, candidiasis is similar to damp accumulation from qi deficiency or qi stagnation that can manifest outwardly in a variety of ways.

Etiology and pathology

The liver, spleen and kidney are the main organs involved in candidiasis.

1. Liver qi stagnation causes the liver to overact on the spleen, leading to spleen deficiency, which causes damp accumulation.
2. Damp accumulation or damp constitution causes either a downward infusion of damp, leading to gastrointestinal problems, or an upward disturbance with heat, involving the lung and upper respiratory system.
3. Lung qi and kidney qi deficiency make one prone to recurrent attacks or lingering candida infections in several areas of the body.

Differentiation and treatment

From the perspective of TCM, candidiasis develops only when disharmony, imbalance, and weakness occur. When the qi (the immune system) is weakened through overwork, stress, or excessive sexual activity, candida flares up and the body cannot control it. In the case of AIDS, *Candida* infection can be life threatening. Candidiasis can be differentiated into three types, with treatment directed toward tonifying qi, transforming damp, spreading liver qi, and restoring balance in the body. U.S. formulas that can be used in all types include *Astra 8* + *Astra C* (HC) and *IM-401* (Pro).

Type	Manifestations	Treatment Principle	Chinese Formula	U.S. Formula and Manufacturer
Liver qi stagnation with damp	Irritability, depression, anger, mood swings, chronic bladder, vaginal and bowel infections, diarrhea or constipation, poor digestion, gas, bloating, dizziness, chronic fatigue worsened with eating, severe PMS; flabby tongue body with thick-coated tongue, wiry or slippery pulse	Move and spread liver qi, transform damp	Classical Formulas: 1. *Xiao Yao San* + *Shen Ling Bai Zhu San* Patent Medicines: 1. *Xiao Yao Wan* + *Shen Ling Bai Zhu Wan* 2. *Qian Jing Zhi Dai Wen*	1. *Break Into a Smile* + *Central Mansion* (TTT) 2. *Bupleurum and Tang Kuei Formula* (GFCH) 3. *Woman's Balance* (HC) 4. *Yellow Xiao Yao San* (ETHP) 5. *PM-637* (Pro) 6. *Harmonize Liver-Spleen* (CMS)
Damp heat disturbance	Chronic infections that flare up with profuse mucus, discharge, and oozing, intestinal cramps, diarrhea, heartburn, rectal itching, food and airborne allergies, athlete's foot, or ringworm, recurrent vaginal or urinary tract infections, prostatitis, feeling light-headed or drunk after small quantities of alcohol or certain foods; sticky, turbid tongue coating, slippery or soft pulse	Transform and eliminate damp phlegm	Classical Formulas: 1. *San Ren Tang* 2. *Er Miao San* 3. *Lian Po Yin* 4. *Gan Lu Xiao Du Dan* Patent Medicines: 1. *Yu Dai Wan* 2. *Qing Qi Hua Tan Wen*	1. *Aquilaria 22* + *Colostroplex* (HC) 2. *Ease the Muscles* + *Clear the Root* (TTT) 3. *A.V.D.* (ETHP) 4. *Purge Phlegm* (CMS) 5. *CY-207* (Pro)
Lung and kidney qi deficiency	Chronic fatigue, extreme sensitivity to environmental exposures, such as cold temperatures, dampness, chemicals, perfumes, smoke, and odors, wandering or chronic, dull muscle and joint aches, symptoms exacerbated by moldy places or damp climates, impotence, low sex drive, no energy to speak, shallow breathing; pale, light-colored tongue body, weak, deep slow pulse	Tonify lung and kidney qi	Classical Formulas: 1. *Liu Jun Zi Tang* + *Bu Fei Tang* + *Liu Wei Di Huang Wan* Patent Medicines: 1. *Xiang Sha Liu Jun Zi Wan* + *Liu Wei Di Huang Wan*	1. *Energy E* (ETHP) 2. *Quiet Contemplative* + *Wise Judge* (Jade and K'an) 3. *Phellostatin* (HC) 4. *Separate Clear and Turbid* + *Soothe the Centre* (TTT) 5. *CY-207* + *IM-401* (Pro) 6. *Harmonize Spleen-Kidney* (CMS)

Cataract

Cataract is a condition affecting the eye in which the lens or lens capsule becomes opaque, resulting in blurry or dim vision. The condition usually affects seniors, occurring predominantly among women, and is thought in most cases to be a natural part of the aging process. Western medicine treats cataracts by removing them surgically when the condition progresses enough to warrant it. In TCM, it is known as *Yuan Yi Nei Zhang*, or "internal screen in the eye."

Etiology and pathology

The liver, kidney, and spleen are the main organs involved in cataract.

1. Liver and kidney deficiency in which blood and essence fail to nourish the eye
2. Spleen qi deficiency in which the source of qi and blood becomes exhausted
3. Liver heat rises and disturbs the clear orifices

Differentiation and treatment

The three types of cataract are differentiated into deficiency two types and excess one type. Treatment should start as soon as possible. Treatment is directed toward nourishing the liver and kidney and promoting the circulation of the eye. U.S. formulas that can be used in all types include *Astra Essence* (HC) and *Gingko Compound* (ETHP).

Type	Manifestations	Treatment Principle	Chinese Formula	U.S. Formula and Manufacturer
Liver and kidney deficiency	Blurred vision, dizziness, tinnitus, weak and achy lower back and knees, frequent and profuse nocturia; pale tongue body, deep weak pulse	Nourish liver and replenish kidney essence	Classical Formulas: 1. *Qi Ju Di Huang Wan* 2. *You Gui Wan* 3. *Ming Mu Di Huang Wan* Patent Medicines: 1. *Qi Ju Di Huang Wan* 2. *You Gui Wan* 3. *Ming Mu Di Huang Wan*	1. *Nine Flavor Tea + Fertile Garden* (HC) 2. *Heaven Age Tea* (ETHP) 3. *Replenish Essence* (CMS) 4. *LI-487* (Pro) 5. *Brighten the Eyes + Strengthen the Root* (TTT) 6. *Quiet Contemplative* (Jade and K'an) 7. *Nourish Essence Formula* (GFCH)

Type	Manifestations	Treatment Principle	Chinese Formula	U.S. Formula and Manufacturer
Spleen qi deficiency	Blurred vision, fatigue, lassitude, sallow complexion, poor appetite, loose stool; pale flabby tongue with thin white coating, slow, thin, weak pulse	Tonify spleen qi	Classical Formulas: 1. *Bu Zhong Yi Qi Tang* 2. *Liu Jun Zi Tang* Patent Medicines: 1. *Bu Zhong Yi Qi Wan* 2. *Xiang Sha Liu Jun Zi Wan*	1. *Arouse Vigor (Jade and K'an)* 2. *Astra 8* (HC) 3. *Tonify Qi and Ease the Muscles* (TTT) 4. *Energy K* (ETHP) 5. *Tonify Qi* (CMS) 6. *Ginseng and Astragalus Formula* (GFCH)
Liver heat	Blurred vision, headaches, excessive eye discharge and pain, red and watery eyes, bitter taste in the mouth, dry mouth and throat; red-edged tongue body with yellow coating, wiry and rapid pulse	Clear liver heat	Classical Formulas: 1. *Shi Jue Ming San* Patent Medicines: 1. *Shi Hu Ye Guang Wan*	1. *Bend Bamboo* (TTT) 2. *Ming Mu Formula* (GFCH) 3. *Clear Vision* (CHC) 4. *G. Plus + Wolfberry Compound* (ETHP)

Chronic Fatigue Syndrome

Chronic fatigue syndrome (CFS), or, as it is now frequently referred to, chronic fatigue immune deficiency syndrome (CFIDS), consists of a series of symptoms including chronic or recurrent fatigue, muscle pains, general depression, headaches, and flulike symptoms, such as sore throat, tender lymph nodes, and chills. Many CFS patients have a history of prolonged stress, repeated infections, and mood swings. CFS often accompanies herpes infection, candidiasis, and hypoglycemia. Lifestyle changes are usually necessary in the treatment of CFS.

Etiology and pathology

TCM tends to view CFS as deficiency syndromes.

1. Qi deficiency
2. Qi and blood deficiency
3. Yin deficiency
4. Yang deficiency
5. Spleen qi and heart blood deficiency

Differentiation and treatment

Treatment is directed toward tonifying qi, blood, yin, and yang. U.S. formulas that can be used in all types and in conjunction with the differentiated formulas are *Astra 8* (HC), *Power Mushrooms* (HC), *EN-261* (Pro), and *Tonify Qi* (CMS).

Type	Manifestations	Treatment Principle	Chinese Formula	U.S. Formula and Manufacturer
Qi deficiency	Chronic fatigue with pale, shiny complexion, lethargy, no spirit, amotivation, puffy looking, weight gain, shortness of breath, depression, sadness; pale, flabby tongue with thin or thick white coating, deep weak or soft pulse	Tonify qi	Classical Formulas: 1. *Si Jun Zi Tang* 2. *Liu Jun Zi Tang* Patent Medicines: 1. *Xiang Sha Liu Jun Zi Tang* 2. *Shen Qi Da Bu Wan*	1. *Move Mountains* (CMS) 2. *EN-261* (Pro) 3. *Prosperous Farmer* (Jade and K'an) 4. *Salvia 10 Formula* (GFCH)
Qi and blood deficiency	Fatigue with pale, dry skin, dry hair, malaise, shortness of breath, dizziness, blurred vision, palpitations, insomnia; pale tongue, weak and thready pulse	Tonify qi and blood	Classical Formulas: 1. *Ba Zhen Tang* 2. *Ren Shen Yang Ying Tang* 3. *Shi Quan Da Bu Tang* Patent Medicines: 1. *Ba Zhen Wan* 2. *Shi Quan Da Bu Wan* 3. *Ren Shen Yang Ying Wan*	1. *Eight Treasures* (HC) 2. *Tonify Blood* (CMS) 3. *Ginseng Nourishing Formula* (GFCH) 4. *EN-261* (Pro) 5. *Women's Precious* (Jade and K'an)

Type	Manifestations	Treatment Principle	Chinese Formula	U.S. Formula and Manufacturer
Yin deficiency	Chronic fatigue with night sweats, flushing, anxiety, five-center burning, low-grade fever, especially in afternoon and evenings, irritable, weight loss, dream-disturbed sleep, insomnia; red or thin tongue body, little coating, thready, rapid pulse	Nourish yin	Classical Formulas: 1. *Liu Wei Di Huang Wan* 2. *Zhi Bai Di Huang Wan* 3. *Da Bu Yin Wan* 4. *Yi Guan Jian* 5. *Zuo Gui Wan* Patent Medicines: 1. *Liu Wei Di Huang Wan* 2. *Zhi Bai Di Huang Wan* 3. *Zuo Gui Wan*	1. *Fertile Garden* (HC) 2. *Nine Flavor Tea* (HC) 3. *Tonify Moisture* (CMS) 4. *R. Plus* (ETHP) 5. *Nourish Essence Formula* (GFCH) 6. *Quiet Contemplative* (Jade and K'an)
Yang deficiency	Chronic fatigue with cold body and limbs, pale complexion, weak low back and lower extremities, lack of sexual interest, impotence, dizziness, tinnitus, frequent urination, nocturia; pale, flabby tongue body, deep, weak pulse	Warm the yang	Classical Formulas: 1. *Jing Gui Shen Qi Wan* 2. *You Gui Wan* 3. *Zan Yu Dan* 4. *Wu Zi Yan Zong Wan* 5. *Da Bu Yuan Jian* Patent Medicines: 1. *Jing Gui Shen Qi Wan* 2. *You Gui Wan* 3. *Gui Ling Ji* 4. *Ge Jie Da Bu Wan*	1. *Rehmannia 8* (HC) 2. *Strengthen Kidney* (CMS) 3. *Dynamic Warrior* (Jade and K'an) 4. *Energy D* (ETHP) 5. *Essential Yang Formula* (GFCH) 6. *MA-511* (Pro)
Spleen qi and heart blood deficiency	Chronic fatigue with gastrointestinal disorders and heart shen disturbance, chronic diarrhea, insomnia, poor appetite, poor digestion, lassitude, general weakness, dream-disturbed sleep with inability to recall dreams, poor memory and concentration, desire to lie down for extended time periods; pale, flabby tongue body with thin or thick white coating, soft, weak pulse	Tonify qi and nourish blood	Classical Formulas: 1. *Gui Pi Tang* Patent Medicines: 1. *Gui Pi Wan*	1. *Gather Vitality* (Jade and K'an) 2. *Shen-Gem* (HC) 3. *Peaceful Spirit Formula* (GFCH) 4. *Energy A* (ETHP) 5. *Calm the Spirit* (TTT)

Common Cold

The common cold is an ailment characterized by nasal obstruction, runny nose, sneezing, coughing, headache, chills, and fever. There are over twenty known viruses that cause the common cold. It is a widespread condition that occurs in all four seasons, especially in winter and spring. In TCM, the pathology of the common cold involves the dysfunction of *wei qi* (defensive qi) and the lungs caused by an invasion of exogenous pathogenic factors.

Etiology and pathology

1. Wind cold: tightening of the skin and muscles, closing of sweat pores and dysfunction of the lung in dispersing
2. Wind heat: disharmony of the lung and defensive qi and dysfunction of the lung in purifying and descending
3. Wind cold with internal damp: obstruction of the clear yang and disharmony of the lung and stomach
4. Cold with weak constitution: loose skin and muscles and reduced body resistance against pathogens
5. Pathogens in between exterior and interior (half exterior and half interior): disharmony of shaoyang qi activities

Differentiation and treatment

Treatment is directed toward dispersing the external pathogen and tonifying the *wei qi*. U.S. formulas that can be used in all types include *Gan Miao Ling* (K'an).

Type	Manifestations	Treatment Principle	Chinese Formula	U.S. Formula and Manufacturer
Wind Cold	Severe aversion to cold, mild fever, anhydrosis (no sweating), headache, soreness, and pain in the limbs, nasal obstruction, thinly running nose, itchy throat, cough, hoarse voice, thin and white sputum, no thirst; thin white tongue coating, superficial and tense pulse	Disperse wind cold to relieve the exterior syndrome and promote dispersing action of the lung qi	Classical Formulas: 1. *Jing Fang Bai Du San*	1. *Prime Rescue* (Jade) 2. *Dispel Invasion* (K'an) 3. *CO-195* (Pro)

Type	Manifestations	Treatment Principle	Chinese Formula	U.S. Formula and Manufacturer
Wind Heat	Severe fever, mild aversion to cold, sweating, headache, cough with yellow and thick sputum, dry, swollen, and sore throat, nasal obstruction with yellow, thick discharge, thirst; red tip and edges of the tongue, thin white or slight yellow coating, superficial and rapid pulse	Disperse wind, clear heat, induce detoxification, promote dispersing function of the lung qi	Classical Formulas: 1. *Yin Qiao San* Patent Medicines: 1. *Yin Chiao Jie Du Wan* 2. *Sang Ju Pian*	1. *Prime Response* (Jade) 2. *Initial Defense* (K'an) 3. *CO-197* (Pro) 4. *Yin Qiao* (K'an) 5. *Yin Chiao Formula* (GFCH) 6. *Zhong Gan Ling* (K'an)
Wind cold with internal damp	Chills, slight fever, headache, fullness or distention in the chest and epigastric area, gastric and abdominal pain, loss of appetite, nausea, vomiting, loose stools or diarrhea; white and greasy tongue coating, moderate or soft pulse	Disperse wind cold to relieve external symptoms, resolve damp, regulate qi; circulate and restore normal action of the middle jiao	Classical Formulas: 1. *Huo Xiang Zheng Qi San* Patent Medicines: 1. *Huo Xiang Zheng Qi Shui*	1. *Prime Relief* (Jade) 2. *Early Comfort* (K'an) 3. *Quiet Digestion* (HC) 4. *Yin Chao Junior* (HC) (for children)
Common cold with weak constitution	Spontaneous perspiration, excessive sweating, easily catch cold, pale complexion; pale tongue body, floating and feeble pulse	Tonify qi, strengthen yang, and relieve external pathogen	Classical Formulas: 1. *Yu Ping Feng San*	1. *IM-401* (Pro) 2. *Jade Windscreen* (K'an) 3. *Jade Screen* (TTT) 4. *Astra-C* (HC) 5. *Herbal Sentinel—Yang* (TTT) 6. *Consolidate Qi* (CMS)
Half exterior and half interior pattern	Alternating fever and chills, dizziness, nausea, chest fullness and congestion; wiry pulse	Harmonize the shaoyang channels	Classical Formulas: 1. *Xiao Chai Hu Tang* Patent Medicines: 1. *Xiao Chai Hu Tang Wan*	1. *Minor Bupleurum* (K'an) 2. *AL-113* (Pro) 3. *Shaoyang Formula* (ETHP)

Conjunctivitis

Conjunctivitis is the inflammation of the conjunctiva, the membrane of the eyelids. It is characterized by red, swollen, congestive, and lacrimating (tearing) eyes and profuse eye discharge and is often referred to as "pinkeye." Chronic conjunctivitis can be caused by excessive use of alcohol; overuse of the eyes; frequent or constant exposure to wind, heat, or poor light; and inadequate sleep. It is known as "red eyes" or "fire eyes" in TCM.

Etiology and pathology

1. Wind heat invasion
2. Liver/gallbladder fire flaring up

Differentiation and treatment

Conjunctivitis is divided into two types. Treatment is directed toward dispersing wind and draining heat and fire from the liver and gallbladder meridians. U.S. formulas that can be used in all types include *A.V.A./hr* (ETHP), *Coptis Relieve Toxicity Formula* (GFCH), and *Windbreaker* (CMS).

Type	Manifestations	Treatment Principle	Chinese Formula	U.S. Formula and Manufacturer
Wind heat	Eye pain, lacrimation, and redness, headache, photophobia, fever, aversion to wind; red tongue tip with thin yellow coating, floating and rapid pulse	Clear heat, disperse wind	Classical Formulas: 1. *Yin Qiao San* 2. *Xie Fei Yin* 3. *Fang Feng Tong Sheng San* Patent Medicines: 1. *Yin Chiao Jie Du Pian* 2. *Fang Feng Tong Sheng Wan*	1. *Yin Chao Jin + New Astra 18 Diet* (HC) 2. *Yin Chiao Formula + Coptis Relieve Toxicity Formula* (GFCH) 3. *Expel Wind-Heat* (TTT) 4. *Prime Response* (Jade) 5. *Initial Defense* (K'an) 6. *Clear Lungs* (CHC) 7. *CO-197* (Pro) 8. *Purge Heat* (CMS)

Type	Manifestations	Treatment Principle	Chinese Formula	U.S. Formula and Manufacturer
Liver/ gallbladder fire	Eye swelling, congestion, redness and pain, sticky yellow eye discharge, bitter taste in the mouth, irritability, feverish sensation, constipation; red tongue body with yellow coating, wiry rapid pulse	Drain the liver/ gallbladder fire	Classical Formulas: 1. *Long Dan Xie Gan Tang* Patent Medicines: 1. *Long Dan Xie Gan Wan*	1. *Coptis Purge Fire* (HC) 2. *Drain Fire* (TTT) 3. *Quell Fire* (Jade and K'an) 4. *R.D.Y.* (ETHP) 5. *Detox Compound* (CHC) 6. *LD-477* (Pro) 7. *Gentiana Drain Fire Formula* (GFCH) 8. *Purge Damp Heat* (CMS)

Constipation

The clinical diagnosis of constipation has two key components. First, the stool is hard and dry and difficult to pass. Second, bowel movements occur infrequently, only every three days or more. The condition may occur as a disease itself or as a symptom of other diseases. Although in TCM constipation is caused mainly by dysfunction of the large intestine in its transportation role, it can also relate to imbalances of the spleen, stomach, and kidney.

Etiology and pathology

1. Excessive yang and retention of heat in the stomach and intestines
2. Irregular emotion and stagnation of qi
3. Deficiency of qi
4. Deficiency of blood
5. Kidney yin deficiency
6. Yang deficiency resulting in yin cold

Differentiation and treatment

U.S. formulas that can be used in all types include *Smooth Response* (K'an and Jade).

Type	Manifestations	Treatment Principle	Chinese Formula	U.S. Formula and Manufacturer
Heat	Dry stool, scanty, dark yellow urine, flushed face, heat sensations in the body, abdominal distention or pain, restlessness, thirst, halitosis; red tongue body, dry yellow coating, slippery rapid pulse	Clear heat, moisten the intestines	Classical Formulas: 1. *Ma Zi Ren Wan*	1. *Gentle Senna* (HC) 2. *HE 349* (Pro)
Qi stagnation	Difficult defecation, distending pain in the hypochondrium and abdomen, distress in the chest and epigastrium, belching, poor appetite; thin, greasy tongue coating, wiry pulse	Promote qi circulation to remove qi stagnation	Classical Formulas: 1. *Liu Mo Tang*	1. *Disperse Qi + Purge Qi* (CMS) 2. *Relaxed Wanderer* (K'an and Jade)
Qi deficiency	Urge to defecate but insufficient force to do so, sweating, shortness of breath during defecation, lassitude after defecation, pale complexion; pale, tender tongue body, thin coating, feeble pulse	Tonify qi, moisten the intestines	Classical Formulas: 1. *Bu Zhong Yi Qi Tang* Patent Medicines: 1. *Bu Zhong Yi Qi Wan* + hemp seed and white honey	1. *Arouse Vigor* (Jade) + hemp seed and white honey *Note*: The above may be used with *Smooth Response* (K'an and Jade).
Blood deficiency	Dry stool, pale complexion, dizziness, blurred vision, heart palpitations, pale lips; pale tongue body, thin and uneven pulse	Tonify blood, moisten dryness	Patent Medicines: 1. *Ren Chang Wan*	1. *Tonify Blood* (CMS) + *Smooth Response* (K'an and Jade)
Yin deficiency	Dry stool, feverish sensation and restlessness, dry mouth, thirst, emaciation, weakness of the low back and knees; red tongue body, scant coating, thin and rapid pulse	Tonify yin, increase body fluid	Patent Medicines:: 1. *Ren Chang Wan + Liu Wei Di Huang Wan*	1. *Smooth Response* (K'an and Jade) + *Quiet Contemplative* (Jade and K'an) 2. *Nine Flavor Tea* (HC)
Yin cold	Difficult defecation, profuse, clear urine, pale complexion, cold extremities, intolerance of cold, preference for warmth, abdominal pain with cold sensation, soreness and pain in lower back; pale tongue body with white coating, deep and slow pulse	Warm yang, relieve stagnation of yin cold	Classical Formulas: 1. *Ji Chuan Jian + Rou Gui*	1. *Dynamic Warrior* (Jade and K'an) 2. *Purge Cold* (CMS) 3. *Po Plus* (ETHP)

Diarrhea

Diarrhea is characterized by increased frequency of bowel movements, loose stools, or, in more severe cases, watery stools. In TCM, it is usually due to disorder of the spleen, stomach, and large and small intestines. It can be caused by invasion of exogenous pathogenic factors, improper diet, emotional stimuli, and deficiency in Zang and Fu organs.

Etiology and pathology

The basic pathogenic changes of diarrhea are dysfunction of the spleen in transformation and transportation and abnormality of the spleen qi in ascending.

1. Exogenous pathogens
   - Damp cold (wind cold)
   - Damp heat (summer heat)
2. Improper diet
3. Irregular emotion
4. Spleen and stomach deficiency
5. Kidney yang deficiency

Differentiation and treatment

U.S. formulas that can be used in all types include *Central Mansion* (TTT).

Type	Manifestations	Treatment Principle	Chinese Formula	U.S. Formula and Manufacturer
Damp cold (wind cold)	Loose stool, or watery diarrhea, abdominal pain and borborygmus, fullness in the epigastric region, poor appetite, aversion to cold, fever, nasal obstruction, headache, general aching; thin white or white greasy tongue coating, soft and moderate pulse	Disperse cold and resolve damp, restore the normal function of the spleen to stop the diarrhea	Classical Formulas: 1. *Huo Xiang Zheng Qi San* Patent Medicines: 1. *Huo Xiang Zheng Qi Wan*	1. *Prime Relief* (Jade) 2. *Early Comfort* (K'an) 3. *Upper Burner: Immune Dynamic* (Jade)

Type	Manifestations	Treatment Principle	Chinese Formula	U.S. Formula and Manufacturer
Damp heat (summer heat)	Diarrhea with abdominal pain, yellow, hot and fetid stool, burning sensation in the anus, restlessness, fever, thirst, scanty urine; red tongue body, yellow greasy coating, rapid and soft pulse or rapid and slippery pulse	Clear heat and resolve damp	Classical Formulas: 1. *Ge Gen Qin Lian Tang* Patent Medicines: 1. *Huang Lian Su Pian* 2. *Xiang Lian Wan*	1. *Copticlear* (K'an) 2. *CoptiDetox* (K'an) 3. *Phellostatin* (HC)
Retention of food	Abdominal pain and borborygmus relieved after bowel movements, diarrhea with fetid stool and undigested food, fullness and distention in the epigastrium and abdomen, belching, acid regurgitation, anorexia; thick, dirty tongue coating or thick, greasy tongue coating, slippery pulse	Promote digestion to remove undigested food	Classical Formulas: 1. *Bao He Wan* Patent Medicines: 1. *Bao He Wan* 2. *Da Shan Zha Wan*	1. *Meal Mover* (CMS) 2. *Quiet Digestion* (HC) 3. *Purge Qi* (CMS)
Disharmony between the liver and spleen	Diarrhea with abdominal pain after depression, anger and stress in mood, fullness and distention in the chest and hypochondriac regions, belching, poor appetite; light red tongue body, wiry pulse	Suppress the liver and strengthen the spleen	Classical Formulas: 1. *Tong Xie Yao Fang*	1. *Harmonize Liver and Spleen* (CMS) *Note: Strengthen Spleen* (CMS) may be added.
Spleen and stomach deficiency	Loose or watery stool with undigested food, aggravated after eating rich and greasy food, anorexia, epigastric distention, sallow complexion, lassitude; pale tongue body, white coating, thready and weak pulse	Tonify the spleen and strengthen the stomach to stop the diarrhea	Classical Formulas: 1. *Li Zhong Tang* 2. *Shen Ling Bai Zhu San* Patent Medicines: 1. *Xiang Sha Liu Jun Zi Wan* 2. *Fu Zi Li Zhong Wan* 3. *Bu Zhong Yi Qi Wan*	1. *Prosperous Farmer* (Jade) 2. *Arouse Vigor* (Jade) 3. *Source Qi* (HC) 4. *Middle Burner: Immune Balance* (Jade)
Kidney yang deficiency	Diarrhea, usually occurring at dawn, with abdominal pain relieved after bowel movements, intolerance of cold, cold extremities, soreness and weakness of the loins and knees; pale tongue body, deep and thin pulse	Warm the kidney, strengthen the spleen, induce astringency to arrest the diarrhea	Patent Formula: 1. *Si Shen Wan* 2. *Fu Zi Li Zhong Wan*	1. *Purge Cold* (CMS) + *Consolidate Qi* (CMS)

Dysmenorrhea

Dysmenorrhea refers to pain in the lower abdomen or lower back before, during, or after menstruation. The pain can be accompanied by nausea, vomiting, restlessness, or cold limbs and, in extreme cases, coma. This condition corresponds to functional dysmenorrhea, membranous dysmenorrhea, endometriosis dysmenorrhea, and inflammatory dysmenorrhea in Western medicine.

Etiology and pathology

1. Qi and blood stagnation
2. Retention of damp cold
3. Accumulation of damp heat
4. Qi and blood deficiency
5. Liver and kidney deficiency

Differentiation and treatment

U.S. formulas that can be used in all types include *Free Flow* (WT) and *PM-637* (Pro).

Type	Manifestations	Treatment Principle	Chinese Formula	U.S. Formula and Manufacturer
Qi and blood stagnation	Pain in the lower abdomen, usually starting before menstruation, unsmooth discharge of menses, scanty volume, dark purple and mixed with clots, distending pain in the lower abdomen, alleviated by passing out the clots, distention in the hypochondriac region and breasts; normal or purple tongue body with purple spots on its edge, wiry or deep wiry pulse	Regulate qi, activate blood circulation, remove stagnation and stop pain	Classical Formulas: 1. *Ge Xia Zhu Yu Tang* Patent Medicines: 1. *Tong Jing Wan* 2. *Yun Nan Bai Yao*	1. *Stir-Field of Elixir* (WT) 2. *Purge Blood* (CMS) 3. *Women's Rhythm* (Jade and K'an) 4. *Crampbark Plus* (HC) 5. *Women's Chamber* (K'an) 6. *Women's Palace* (Jade)

Type	Manifestations	Treatment Principle	Chinese Formula	U.S. Formula and Manufacturer
Damp cold	Cold sensation and pain or colicky pain in the lower abdomen before or during menstruation that can be relieved by warmth, scanty, dark menses with clots, unsmooth discharge of menses, intolerance of cold, loose stool; white sticky tongue coating, deep tense pulse	Warm channels and collaterals, disperse cold, resolve dampness, and relieve pain	Classical Formulas: 1. *Wen Jing Tang + Fu zi, Ai ye, Xiao hui xiang* 2. *Shao Fu Zhu Yu Tang* Patent Medicines: 1. *Ai Fu Nuan Gong Wan*	1. *Women's Journey* (K'an and Jade) 2. *Warm the Menses* (WT) 3. *Warm the Mansion* (WT)
Damp heat	Abdominal pain with burning sensation, aggravated by pressure, distending pain in the lumbrosacral region, pain before menstruation or worse after arrival of menses, dark red thick menses with clots, thick yellow leukorrhea, scanty yellow urine; red tongue body with yellow and sticky coating, wiry and rapid pulse or soft and rapid pulse	Clear damp heat, remove stagnation, and stop pain	Classical Formulas: 1. *Qing Re Tiao Xue Tang + Hong Teng, Bai Jiang Cao, Yi Yi Ren* 2. *Long Dan Xie Gan Tang* Patent Medicines: 1. *Long Dan Xie Gan Wan*	1. *Drain Redness* (WT) 2. *Quell Fire* (K'an and Jade) 3. *Gentiana Drain Fire Formula* (GFCH)
Qi and blood deficiency	Lingering, dull lower abdominal pain with hollow or bearing-down sensation during or after menstruation, alleviated by pressure, pale and thin menses, pale complexion, fatigue; pale tongue body, thready and weak pulse	Tonify qi and blood	Classical Formulas: 1. *Sheng Yu Tang* Patent Medicines: 1. *Ren Shen Yang Rong Wan*	1. *Women's Precious* (K'an and Jade) 2. *Precious Sea* (WT) 3. *Eight Treasures* (HC)
Liver and kidney deficiency	Dull lower abdominal pain after menstruation, pale scanty menses, soreness and weakness of the lumbar region, dizziness, tinnitus; pale tongue body, thin coating, deep and thin pulse	Tonify the liver and kidney, regulate and strengthen chong and ren	Classical Formulas: 1. *Tiao Gan Tang* Patent Medicines: 1. *Qi Ju Di Huang Wan*	1. *Unicorn Pearl* (WT)

Ear Infection

Ear infection (*otitis media*) is an acute or chronic inflammation of the *auris media* (middle ear). The most common form of ear infection, seen mostly in children, is characterized by otopyorrhea (excessive ear discharge) and ear pain. TCM refers to *otitis media* as *ting er*, or "purulent ear."

Etiology and pathology

The shaoyang meridians are mainly involved in otitis media.

1. Wind heat invasion
2. Gallbladder damp heat causing upward disturbance
3. Yin fluid deficiency leading to inadequate nourishment

Differentiation and treatment

There are usually two types differentiated: acute (excess) and chronic (deficiency). Treatment is directed toward clearing heat and expelling pus from the ear for the acute type and moistening the shaoyang, liver, and kidney meridians for the chronic type. U.S. formulas that can be used in all types include *Ear Clear* (CHC) and *Yin Chao Junior* (HC).

Type	Manifestations	Treatment Principle	Chinese Formula	U.S. Formula and Manufacturer
Acute type from wind heat or gallbladder damp heat	Sudden onset, throbbing pain in the ear, hearing impaired, possible fever, chills, headache, dizziness; rapid, floating pulse; possible yellow purulent discharge within a few days of onset due to eardrum rupture; red tongue with yellow coating, rapid, slippery pulse	Clear heat and expel pus	Classical Formulas: 1. *Yin Qiao San* 2. *Man Jing Zi San* 3. *Long Dan Xie Gan Tang* 4. *Xian Fang Huo Ming Yin* Patent Medicines: 1. *Yin Chiao Jie Du Pian* 2. *Long Dan Xie Gan Wan*	1. *Yin Chao Jin* + *Isatis Gold* (HC) 2. *Prime Response* + *Quell Fire* (Jade) 3. *Initial Defense* + *Quell Fire* (K'an) 4. *Children's Herbal Sentinal* + *Expel Wind Heat* (TTT) (initial stage) 5. *Expel Wind Heat* + *Drain Fire* (TTT) (severe cases) 6. *Isatis Compound* (ETHP) 7. *Purge Damp Heat* (CMS)

Type	Manifestations	Treatment Principle	Chinese Formula	U.S. Formula and Manufacturer
Chronic type—yin fluid deficiency	Lingering or recurrent attacks of *otitis media*, continuous thin scanty purulent discharge from ear, dizziness, impaired hearing, tinnitus, exacerbation by cold/flu or swimming, possible lassitude, mild fever; pale, dry tongue, deep thready pulse	Nourish yin fluids	Classical Formulas: 1. *Zhi Bai Di Huang Wan* 2. *Zuo Gui Wan* Patent Medicines: 1. *Zhi Bai Di Huang Wan* 2. *Zuo Gui Wan*	1. *Nine Flavor Tea + Astra C* (HC) 2. *Ease the Journey—Yin* (TTT) 3. *Strengthen Kidney* (CMS) 4. *Energy L + Sheng Mai San Plus* (ETHP) 5. *Rehmannia and Scrophularia Formula* (GFCH) 6. *Temper Fire* (Jade and K'an)

Early Menstrual Cycle

A menstrual period that occurs seven or more days earlier than normal is considered an early menstrual cycle.

Etiology and Pathology

1. Qi deficiency
2. Blood heat—excess
   - excessive yang and blood heat
   - liver qi stagnation and blood heat
3. Blood heat—deficient

Differentiation and treatment

U.S. formulas that can be used in all types include *Penetrating Wind Vessel* (WT) and *Full Circle* (CHC).

Type	Manifestations	Treatment Principle	Chinese Formula	U.S. Formula and Manufacturer
Qi deficiency	Early menstrual cycle with profuse, light-colored, thin menses, lassitude, shortness of breath, poor appetite, loose stool; pale tongue body, thready and weak pulse; palpitations, poor sleep and dream disturbed sleep in some cases	Tonify qi, invigorate the spleen, control the blood, and regulate the menstruation	Classical Formulas: 1. *Bu Zhong Yi Qi Tang* 2. *Gui Pi Tang* Patent Medicines: 1. *Bu Zhong Yi Qi Wan* 2. *Gui Pi Wan*	1. *Arouse Vigor* (K'an and Jade) 2. *Source Qi* (HC) 3. *Ginseng and Astragalus Formula* (GFCH) 4. *Gather Vitality* (K'an and Jade)
Blood heat—yang heat	Early cycle with profuse scarlet or purplish red colored, thick menses, restlessness, feeling of suffocation, flushed face, dry mouth, scanty yellow urine, premenstrual constipation; red tongue body, yellow coating, rapid pulse	Clear heat from the blood and regulate the Chong and Ren channels	Classical Formulas: 1. *Qing Jing San* 2. *Bao Yin Jian*	1. *Cool the Menses* (WT) 2. *Clear Empty-Heat and Cool the Menses* (WT)
Blood heat—liver qi stagnation	Early menstrual cycle with profuse or scanty menses, purplish red, mixed with blood clots; fullness in the chest or hypochondrium, distending pain in the lower abdomen, dysphoria, irritability, bitter taste in the mouth, dry throat; red tongue body, thin and yellow coating, wiry and rapid pulse	Clear heat from the blood and move liver qi	Classical Formulas: 1. *Dan Zhi Xiao Yao San*	1. *Woman's Balance* (HC) 2. *PM-637* (Pro) 3. *Free Flow* (WT) 4. *Free and Easy Wanderer Plus* (GFCH) *Note:* Above products may be used in combination with *Cool the Menses* (WT).
Blood heat—deficient heat	Early menstrual cycle with menses profuse or scanty, red, and thick; flushed cheeks, hot sensation in the palms and soles; red tongue body, scanty coating, thin and rapid pulse	Clear deficient heat	Classical Formulas: 1. *Liang Di Tang* Patent Medicines 1. *Zhi Bai Di Huang Wan*	1. *Temper Fire* (K'an and Jade)

Eczema

Eczema is a skin condition characterized by itching red areas with weeping vesicles. It may progress to the point of scaling and pigmentation. In TCM, eczema's name varies with its location on the body. When it manifests on infants' faces, it is called "milk ringworm." In the ear, it is called simply "ear rash," and in the genital area, "kidney wind." If it spreads all over, it is known as "blood wind" or "millet sore."

Etiology and pathology

Eczema can be divided into two types: acute and chronic.

1. Acute eczema is caused by wind damp heat lingering in the skin-muscle layer that blocks the skin-muscles and related collaterals.
2. Chronic eczema comes from wind dry due to blood and fluid deficiency or blood heat, in which the skin fails to be nourished by the blood and fluids.

Differentiation and treatment

Eczema is generally characterized by a variety of shapes and sizes of skin lesions, symmetrical distribution, itching, recurrence, and a tendency to become chronic. U.S. formulas that can be used in all types include *Skin Cleanser* (LLHP) and *SK-741* (Pro).

Type	Manifestations	Treatment Principle	Chinese Formula	U.S. Formula and Manufacturer
Acute stage—damp heat	Red, itchy skin at onset that progresses quickly to rash with small vesicles; with scratching, weeping lesions appear, abdominal pain, diarrhea, or constipation, scanty urine, headache, fever; yellow or yellow sticky tongue coating, floating rapid or rolling rapid pulse	Disperse wind damp and clear heat	Classical Formulas: 1. *Er Miao San* 2. *Bei Xie Shen Shi Tang* 3. *Long Dan Xie Gan Tang* Patent Medicines: 1. *Long Dan Xie Gan Wan* 2. *Chuan Shan Jia Kang Shi Du Wan*	1. *Skin Balance* (HC) 2. *ZiCao Compound* (ETHP) 3. *Golden Balm* (ETHP) (topical use) 4. *Coptis Relieve Toxicity Formula* (GFCH) 5. *Clear Lustre* (TTT) 6. *Clear Skin* (CHC) 7. *Phlogisticlean* (CMS) 8. *Quell Fire* (Jade and K'an) 9. *CY-207* (Pro)

Type	Manifestations	Treatment Principle	Chinese Formula	U.S. Formula and Manufacturer
Chronic stage—blood/fluid deficiency	Recurrence of eczema, affected areas pigmenting darker or brown; rough, thick, and itchy skin, skin crusty and crumbling off; pale tongue body with thin white coating; thready pulse	Nourish blood and fluid, disperse wind	Classical Formulas: 1. *Si Wu Xiao Feng Yin* 2. *Dang Gui Yin Zi*	1. *Eight Treasures* (HC) 2. *Glorious Sea* (TTT) 3. *Energy C* (ETHP) 4. *Tonify Moisture* (CMS) 5. *Eight Immortals Formula* (GFCH)

Gastric Pain (Stomachache)

Gastric (or epigastric) pain is a common symptom manifested by frequent pain over the epigastric region. In ancient times, it was mistakenly called cardiac pain because the painful area is often close to the center of the chest. It is different, however, from true cardiac pain. Gastric pain is commonly seen in acute and chronic gastritis, gastric or duodenal ulcers, gastroneurosis, and gastric cancer in Western medicine, so the treatment discussed below can be used for these diseases.

Etiology and pathology

In TCM, the basic pathology of gastric pain is disorder of the stomach qi in descending, which leads to qi obstruction in the epigastrium.

1. Invasion of the stomach by cold
2. Injury of the stomach due to irregular meals
3. Liver qi attacking the stomach
4. Accumulation of fire in the stomach
5. Retention of the blood stasis in the stomach
6. Deficiency of the spleen and stomach

Differentiation and treatment

U.S. formulas that can be used in all types include *Shu Gan* (HC).

Type	Manifestations	Treatment Principle	Chinese Formula	U.S. Formula and Manufacturer
Stomach cold	Sudden onset of gastric pain, alleviated by warmth, intolerance of cold, preference for warmth, absence of thirst or thirst with desire for drinking hot fluid; white and thin coating on tongue, wiry or tense pulse	Disperse cold and warm the stomach	Classical Formulas: 1. *Liang Fu Wan* Patent Medicines: 1. *Liang Fu Wan*	1. *Purge Cold* (CMS)
Retention of food	Distending pain in the epigastrium, aggravated by pressure, belching with fetid odor, acid regurgitation, or vomiting with undigested food, anorexia; thick, greasy tongue coating, slippery pulse	Promote digestion to remove undigested food	Classical Formulas: 1. *Bao He Wan* Patent Medicines: 1. *Bao He Wan* 2. *Da Shan Zha Wan*	1. *Meal Mover* (CMS) 2. *Purge Qi* (CMS)
Liver qi attacking the stomach	Paroxysmal distending pain in the epigastrium, radiating to the hypochondriac regions, usually occurring after drastic emotional changes, frequent belching; thin, white tongue coating, deep and wiry pulse	Soothe the liver and relieve obstruction of stomach qi	Classical Formulas: 1. *Chai Hu Shu Gan San* Patent Medicines: 1. *Shu Gan He Wei Wan* 2. *Shu Gan Wan*	1. *Break into A Smile* (TTT) 2. *Disperse Qi* (CMS)
Stomach fire	Paroxysmal pain with burning sensation, foul belching, acid regurgitation, restlessness, hot temper, thirst, bitter taste in the mouth, dry stool, dark yellow urine; wiry and rapid pulse	Purge the stomach fire	Classical Formulas: 1. *Zuo Jin Wan* Patent Medicines: 1. *Zuo Jin Wan*	1. *GI-335* (Pro) 2. *GI-337* (Pro) *Note:* The above can be used with *PM-637* (Pro), *Woman's Balance* (HC), or *Relaxed Wanderer* (Jade and K'an).

Type	Manifestations	Treatment Principle	Chinese Formula	U.S. Formula and Manufacturer
Stagnation of blood	Fixed, sharp pain in the epigastrium, aggravated by pressure; in severe cases, vomiting blood, bloody stool; dark red tongue body with purple spots, uneven pulse	Promote blood circulation to remove blood stasis	Classical Formulas: 1. *Shi Xiao San* + *Dan Shen Yin* + *Gan cao, Da huang* Patent Medicines: 1. *Yuan Hu Zhi Tong Pian*	1. *VA-841* (Pro) + *Break Into a Smile* (TTT) 2. *Purge Blood* (BOP) 3. *Invigorate the Collaterals* (K'an)
Stomach yin deficiency	Dull pain in the epigastrium, sometimes with burning sensation, dry mouth and throat with desire to drink, dry stool or constipation; red tongue body with scanty coating, thready and rapid pulse	Nourish stomach yin and clear deficient fire	Classical Formulas: 1. *Yi Wei Tang* 2. *Mai Men Dong Tang*	1. *Jade Spring* (TTT) 2. *Tonify Moisture* (CMS)
Deficient cold of the spleen and stomach	Dull, cold pain, preference for warmth and pressure, aggravated when hungry and alleviated after meal, vomiting clear or sputumlike fluid, poor appetite, lassitude, cold limbs, loose stools; pale tongue body, weak or slow pulse	Warm the middle jiao and invigorate the spleen	Classical Formulas: 1. *Huang Qi Jian Zhong Tang* Patent Medicines: 1. *Fu Zi Li Zhong Wan*	1. *Purge Cold* (CMS) 2. *New Astra 8* (HC)

Glaucoma

Glaucoma is an eye condition in which the fluid balance of the eyeball is upset, with more fluid staying in than exiting. This results in a painful buildup of fluid in the eyeball that creates pressure, leading to impaired vision. If untreated, the pressure can cause atrophy of the optic nerve and result in blindness. Patients often report seeing halos around lights in earlier stages. Onset can be rapid and acute or slow and chronic. TCM refers to glaucoma as *Qing Feng Nei Zhang*, or "green wind internal blockage."

Etiology and pathology

The liver, kidney, and spleen are the main organs involved in glaucoma.

1. Emotional stress, worries, and anger lead to liver qi stagnation which turns to liver fire.
2. Spleen deficiency results in damp phlegm accumulation which transforms to fire rising that affects the eye.
3. True yin gets consumed internally leading to empty fire rising which impairs the eyes.

Differentiation and treatment

Because glaucoma can result in blindness, early treatment intervention is especially important. Treatment is directed toward clearing heat, eliminating damp phlegm, and nourishing yin. U.S. formulas that can be used in all types include *A.V.C.* (ETHP).

Type	Manifestations	Treatment Principle	Chinese Formula	U.S. Formula and Manufacturer
Liver qi stagnation with liver fire	Distending pain in the head and eye, accompanied by irritability, hypochondriac pain, and distension, bitter taste in the mouth, nausea; red tongue body with yellow coating, thready or wiry pulse	Spread and move liver qi, clear heat	Classical Formulas: 1. *Dan Zhi Xiao Yao San* Patent Medicines: 1. *Xiao Yao Wan*	1. *G. Plus* (ETHP) 2. *Smooth Passage* (TTT) 3. *Woman's Balance* (HC) 4. *Relaxed Wanderer* (Jade and K'an) 5. *Free and Easy Wanderer Plus* (GFCH) 6. *PM-637* (Pro)
Phlegm fire rising	Hot pain in the eye, blurred vision, dizziness, irritability, palpitations, poor appetite, profuse sputum, congestion in the chest and epigastrium, nausea, bitter taste in the mouth; red tongue body with yellow, greasy coating, wiry, rapid, slippery pulse	Clear heat and eliminate phlegm	Classical Formulas: 1. *Huang Lian Wen Dan Tang* Patent Medicines: 1. *Huang Lian Shang Qing Pian*	1. *Clear Phlegm* (HC) 2. *CR-201* (Pro) 3. *PhL-II* (ETHP) 4. *Lucid Clarity* (Jade) 5. *Lucid Channel* (K'an) 6. *Anxiety Calm* (LLHP) 7. *Purge Phlegm* (CMS)

Type	Manifestations	Treatment Principle	Chinese Formula	U.S. Formula and Manufacturer
Liver and kidney yin deficiency with empty fire	Prolonged illness, decreased vision, blurred vision, no spirit in the eye, distending eye pain, slightly enlarged pupil, reports of halos around lights, tinnitus, insomnia, poor memory, weak and achy low back and knees, heat sensations in the palms and soles, symptoms exacerbated by exertion; red tongue body with little or no coating, rapid, thready, deep weak pulse	Tonify liver and kidney yin	Classical Formulas: 1. *Qi Ju Di Huang Wan* Patent Medicines: 1. *Qi Ju Di Huang Wan*	1. *Ming Mu Formula* (GFCH) 2. *Wolfberry Compound* (ETHP) 3. *Replenish Essence* (CMS) 4. *Brighten the Eyes* (TTT) 5. *Astra Essence + Nine Flavor Tea* (HC)

Headache

Headache is a common clinical symptom encountered in many acute and chronic diseases. This section discusses headache only as the predominant symptom. Headache as an accompanying symptom in the presentation of a specific disease, which disappears when the disease is cured, is not addressed in this section. According to TCM, all the yang meridians of the hands and feet meet at the head, and the qi and blood of the five Zang organs and six Fu organs all flow upward to the head. The basic pathogenic changes of headache are obstruction of qi in the meridians, derangement of qi and blood in the head, and malnourishment of the brain caused by attacks of exogenous pathogenic factors as well as endogenous injury.

Etiology and pathology

Exogenous Pathogenic Factors

1. Invasion of wind cold
2. Invasion of wind heat
3. Invasion of wind damp

Endogenous Factors

1. Upsurge of liver yang
2. Deficiency of the kidney
3. Deficiency of the ying blood
4. Damp phlegm stagnation
5. Blood stagnation

Differentiation and treatment

U.S. formulas that can be used in all types include *HA-341* (Pro).

Type	Manifestations	Treatment Principle	Chinese Formula	U.S. Formula and Manufacturer
Wind cold	Headache occurring on exposure to wind cold, paroxysmal pain extending to the nape of the neck and upper back, aversion to wind and cold, no thirst; thin white tongue coating, floating or floating and tight pulse	Disperse wind cold to relieve the headache	Classical Formulas: 1. *Chuan Xiong Cha Tiao San* Patent Medicines: 1. *Chuan Xiong Cha Tiao Wan*	1. *HA-341* (Pro) 2. *Head-Q* (HC) *Note:* Combine with *Prime Rescue* (Jade) or *Dispel Invasion* (K'an) or *CO-195* (Pro) to increase dispersing of wind cold. Combine with *PA-621* (Pro) for rigidity and pain in the nape and the back.
Wind heat	Distending or throbbing headache, fever, aversion to wind, flushed face, bloodshot eyes, thirst with desire to drink, dry stool, yellow urine; slightly red tongue body, thin yellow coating, floating and rapid pulse	Disperse wind and clear heat to stop headache	Classical Formulas: 1. *Xiong Zhi Shi Gao Tang*. Patent Medicines: 1. *Sang Ju Pian* + *Yin Chiao Jie Du Wan*	1. *Initial Defense* (K'an) 2. *Prime Response* (Jade) *Note:* Add *Angelica Dahuricae* (Bai Zhi) to strengthen the action of stopping pain.
Wind damp	Headache with a feeling of the head wrapped up, heavy sensation in the body, anorexia, fullness in the chest, dysuria, loose stool; white and greasy tongue coating, soft pulse	Disperse wind and resolve damp	Classical Formulas: 1. *Qiang Huo Shen Shi Tang* Patent Medicines: 1. *Jiu Wei Qiang Huo Wan* 2. *Huo Xiang Zheng Qi Wan*	1. *HA-341*((Pro) + *Prime Relief* (Jade)

Type	Manifestations	Treatment Principle	Chinese Formula	U.S. Formula and Manufacturer
Liver yang hyperactivity	Headache, blurred vision, dizziness, irritability, hypochondriac pain, flushed face, bitter taste in the mouth; red tongue body, thin yellow coating, wiry and forceful pulse	Calm liver and subdue hyperactivity of liver yang	Classical Formulas: 1. *Tian Ma Gou Teng Yin* Patent Medicines: 1. *Jiang Ya Ping Pian* 2. *Du Zhong Wan*	1. *New Gastrodia Relieve Wind Formula* (HC) 2. *HB-345* (Pro) 3. *Purge Internal Wind* (CMS) 4. *Green Tiger: Water Create Wood* (Jade) *Note:* Add *Quell Fire* (Jade) for liver fire. Add U.S. equivalents of *Liu Wei Di Huang Wan* for presence of kidney yin deficiency
Kidney yin deficiency	Hollow headache, dizziness, soreness and weakness of the loins and knees, lassitude, nocturnal emission, leukorrhea, tinnitus, poor sleep; red tongue body with scanty coating, thin weak pulse	Nourish yin and tonify the kidney	Classical Formulas: 1. *Da Bu Yuan Jian* Patent Medicines: 1. *Zuo Gui Wan* 2. *Qi Ju Di Huang Wan* 3. *Liu Wei Di Huang Wan* (*Six Flavor Rehmannia Pill*)	1. *Quiet Contemplative* (Jade and K'an 2. *Strengthen Kidney* (CMS) 3. *Nine Flavor Tea* (HC) *Note:* For kidney yang deficiency use *Rehmannia 8* (HC) or *Dynamic Warrior* (Jade)
Blood deficiency	Headache accompanied by dizziness, palpitation, general lassitude, pale complexion; pale tongue body, thin and white coating, thready and weak pulse	Tonify blood	Classical Formulas: 1. *Si Wu Tang*	1. *Women's Precious* (Jade and K'an) 2. *Tonify Blood* (CMS) 3. *Eight Treasures* (HC)
Damp phlegm stagnation	Headache with heavy sensation, dizziness, fullness and distention in the chest and epigastrium, nausea, vomiting sputum; white greasy tongue coating, slippery or wiry and slippery pulse	Resolve phlegm and induce qi downward	Classical Formulas: 1. *Ban Xia Bai Zhu Tian Ma Tang* Patent Medicines: 1. *Tian Ma Tou Tong Wan*	1. *Lucid Channel* (K'an) 2. *Lucid Clarity* (Jade) 3. *Purge Phlegm* (CMS) 4. *Clear the Soul* (TTT)

Type	Manifestations	Treatment Principle	Chinese Formula	U.S. Formula and Manufacturer
Blood stagnation	Lingering headache that is prickling and fixed in nature, traumatic injury; purple tongue body, thin and white coating, thready or thready and uneven pulse	Promote blood circulation to remove blood stasis	Classical Formulas: 1. *Tong Qiao Huo Xue Tang* Patent Medicines: 1. *Yuan Hu Zhi Tong Pian* 2. *Pian Tou Tong Wan*	1. *Invigorate the Collaterals* (K'an)

Heart Disease

Heart disease is the leading cause of death in the United States among both men and women. Because in TCM, outward signs and symptoms reflect internal states, heart disease demonstrating the outward symptom of pain is discussed here among the many subcategories of cardiopathy. More specifically, coronary artery disease (CAD), an ischemic cardiopathy in which the coronary arteries become hard and occluded, is considered. TCM refers to this disease as "chest Bi" or "genuine heart pain." Clinical studies suggest that TCM is highly effective in treating heart disease.

Etiology and pathology

Research indicates that the main causes of CAD include poor diet, obesity, stress, mental fatigue, lack of joy, diabetes, hypertension, hypothyroidism, and smoking. The TCM pathology is as follows:

1. Qi and blood stagnation in the heart
2. Damp phlegm blockage in the chest
3. Cold accumulation in the heart meridian from kidney yang deficiency
4. Qi and yin deficiency which leads to a loss of nourishment and heart power

Differentiation and treatment

CAD can be differentiated into four types according to its manifestations, tongue picture, pulse, and constitution. Typical manifestations include palpitations, chest fullness, shortness of breath, cardiac pain, irregular heartbeat, sweating, dizziness, vertigo, stiff tongue and lips, and angina. Treatment focuses on moving qi and blood. U.S. formulas that can be used in all types include *Flavonex* (HC).

Type	Manifestations	Treatment Principle	Chinese Formula	U.S. Formula and Manufacturer
Heart qi and blood stagnation	Localized cardiac twinge or sharp pain, precipitated and exacerbated by exposure to cold temperature, episode intensity increases over time, chest stuffiness, palpitations, shortness of breath; purple-red or spotted purple tongue body with thin coating, choppy, wiry, knotted or intermittent pulse	Move qi and blood, alleviate pain	Classical Formulas: 1. *Dan Shen Yin* + *Tao Hong Si Wu Tang* Patent Medicines: 1. *Fu Fang Dan Shen Pian* 2. *Tian Qi San*	1. *Red Stirring* (TTT) 2. *Women's Palace* (Jade) 3. *Invigorate the Collaterals* (K'an) 4. *Q.B.A.* (ETHP) 5. *VA-841* (Pro) 6. *Disperse Blood* (CMS) 7. *Cinnamon and Poria Formula* (GFCH) 8. *Invigorate QB* (CHC)
Damp phlegm obstruction	Chest stuffiness and pain, overweight, fatigue, heavy feeling all over the body, anorexia, nausea, vomiting mucus; flabby tongue body with thick greasy or sticky tongue coating, slippery, forceful pulse	Dispel obstruction, transform phlegm damp	Classical Formulas: 1. *Wen Dan Tang* 2. *Kuan Xiong Wan* Patent Medicines: 1. *Su He Xiang Wan* 2. *Er Chen Wan*	1. *Clear Phlegm* (HC) 2. *Limpid Sea* (TTT) 3. *Salvia 10 Formula* (GFCH) 4. *Lucid Channel* (K'an) 5. *Lucid Clarity* (Jade) 6. *PhL II* (ETHP) 7. *Purge Phlegm* (CMS)
Cold accumulation	Abrupt onset of cardiac pain, worse with exposure to cold, may radiate to upper back, shortness of breath, palpitations, cold extremities, weak and achy low back and knees; pale tongue body with thin white coating, deep wiry or irregular pulse	Warm yang, move blood, stop pain	Classical Formulas: 1. *Gua Lou Jiao Bai Gui Zhi Tang* 2. *Jin Gui Shen Qi Wan* 3. *You Gui Wan* Patent Medicines: 1. *Jin Gui Shen Qi Wan* 2. *You Gui Wan*	1. *Virility Tablets* (HC) 2. *Energy D* (ETHP) 3. *Purge Cold* (CMS) 4. *Strengthen the Root* (TTT) 5. *Dynamic Warrior* (Jade and K'an)

Type	Manifestations	Treatment Principle	Chinese Formula	U.S. Formula and Manufacturer
Qi and yin deficiency	Dull cardiac pain, shortness of breath, palpitations, spontaneous sweating, night sweats, lassitude, reluctance to talk, dry mouth; thin tongue coating, thready or wiry, irregular pulse	Replenish qi and nourish yin	Classical Formulas: 1. *Sheng Mai San* Patent Medicines: 1. *Fu Fang Wu Wei Zi Pian*	1. *Wise Judge* (Jade and K'an) 2. *Sheng Mai San Plus* (ETHP) 3. *Strengthen Heart + Harmonize Heart-Lung* (CMS) 4. *Sheng Mai San* (LLHP) 5. *Herbal Sentinel-Yin* (TTT) 6. *Heavenly Emperor's Formula* (GFCH) 7. *Marrow Plus* (HC)

Hemorrhoids

Hemorrhoids are enlarged or varicose veins that occur inside or just outside the rectum. Varying degrees of pain, itching, and pressure can accompany hemorrhoids. Bleeding occurs if the external hemorrhoid is ruptured. Hemorrhoids are considered stagnant qi and blood in TCM, which attributes hemorrhoids to exertion, stress, excessive sexual activities, excessive intake of spicy foods or alcohol, prolonged sitting, constipation, or diarrhea.

Etiology and pathology

1. Spleen qi deficiency or sinking
2. Damp heat of the large intestine
3. Liver qi and blood stagnation

Differentiation and treatment

Hemorrhoids can be differentiated into three types and can be treated topically and internally. Treatment is directed toward moving qi, invigorating the blood flow, and transforming blood stasis and damp accumulation. Formulas common to all types are *Fel Ursi Ointment*, *Ma Yin Long Zhi Chuang Gao*, and *Zhi Wan*, all to be applied topically.

Type	Manifestations	Treatment Principle	Chinese Formula	U.S. Formula and Manufacturer
Spleen qi deficiency and sinking	External hemorrhoids, rectal prolapse, slight pain or downward pressure sensation, slight bleeding possible, poor appetite, fatigue, sallow complexion, diarrhea or loose stool; pale, flabby tongue body with thin white coating, deep, frail pulse	Tonify and raise spleen qi, stop bleeding	Classical Formulas: 1. *Bu Zhong Yi Qi Tang* Patent Medicines: 1. *Bu Zhong Yi Qi Wan*	1. *Source Qi* (HC) 2. *Energy K* (ETHP) 3. *Soothe the Center* (TTT) 4. *Prosperous Farmer* (Jade and K'an) 5. *Ginseng and Astragalus Formula* (GFCH) 6. *Tonify Qi* (CMS) 7. *EN-261* (Pro)
Large intestine damp heat	Bleeding hemorrhoids with burning sensations, frequent and urgent bowel movements, often accompanied by either constipation or foul-smelling diarrhea, halitosis; red tongue body with sticky yellow coating, slippery, rapid pulse	Transform damp, clear heat	Classical Formulas: 1. *Huai Hua San* 2. *Bai Tou Weng Tang* 3. *Ge Gen Qin Lian Tang*	1. *Formula H* (HC) 2. *Wu Hua Formula* (GFCH) 3. *D.U. Compound* (ETHP)
Liver qi and blood stagnation	Recurrent hemorrhoids with emotional stress, dark red or purple hemorrhoids, depression, anger, frequent belching, bloating, flank pain; dark red or purple tongue body, wiry pulse	Move liver qi and blood	Classical Formulas: 1. *Chai Hu Shu Gan San* 2. *Shi Xiao San* 3. *Xiao Yao San* Patent Medicines: 1. *Shu Gan Wan* 2. *Xiao Yao Wan*	1. *Bupleurum Entangled Qi Formula* (HC) 2. *Freeing the Moon* (TTT) 3. *Energy E* (ETHP) 4. *Free and Easy Wanderer Plus* (GFCH) 5. *Relaxed Wanderer* (Jade and K'an)

Herpes Simplex and Herpes Zoster

All types of herpes are inflammatory skin diseases caused by a herpes virus; they manifest as small vesicles on the skin. Although there are many subtypes of herpes, only herpes simplex and herpes zoster are considered here. Herpes simplex is characterized by red, painful, itchy skin outbreaks in the genital area, or along the liver meridian in TCM, and on the neck and face including the lips and mouth, corresponding to the stomach and large intestine meridians in TCM. Herpes zoster usually occurs around the waist along the Dai meridian, but can appear along the jaw and neck as well. Both types of herpes are affected by stress, diet, and exertion. In general, foods to avoid are coffee, alcohol, and chocolate, as well as hot or overly pungent herbs and spices, such as ginger, garlic, onions, and pepper. Seafood and dairy products should also be avoided.

Etiology and pathology

Heat toxin is the chief causative factor; diet and emotions are catalysts.

1. Liver qi stagnation with damp heat
2. Dai meridian damp heat
3. Wind fire with qi deficiency

Differentiation and treatment

Treatment in TCM is directed toward eliminating toxic heat and alleviating the skin lesions. U.S formulas common to all types include *Astra Isatis* (HC), *White Flower* (ETHP), and *Herpecream* (LLHP) (topical application).

Type	Manifestations	Treatment Principle	Chinese Formula	U.S. Formula and Manufacturer
Liver qi stagnation with damp heat	Outbreaks of lesions in the genital area, lips, or mouth, accompanied and triggered by emotional stress, itching, redness, pain, irritability; red or dark red tongue body with sticky yellow coating, rapid, wiry pulse	Move liver qi, eliminate damp heat toxin	Classical Formulas: 1. *Long Dan Xie Gan Tang* 2. *Dan Zhi Xiao Yao San* Patent Medicines: 1. *Long Dan Xie Gan Wan*	1. *Coptis Purge Fire* (HC) 2. *Quell Fire* (Jade) 3. *Lotus Balm* (ETHP) (topical application) 4. *Gentiana Drain Fire Formula* (GFCH) 5. *Purge Damp Heat* (CMS) 6. *LD-477* (Pro)

Type	Manifestations	Treatment Principle	Chinese Formula	U.S. Formula and Manufacturer
Dai meridian damp heat	Red, painful, itchy vesicles at waist area, irritability, anxiety; red tongue body with greasy yellow coating, rapid, slippery pulse	Clear and transform damp heat from Dai	Classical Formulas: 1. *Zhi Zi Qing Gan Tang* 2. *Wei Ling Tang*	1. *Drain Dampness + Phellostatin* (HC) 2. *Five Detox* (LLHP) 3. *Coptis Relieve Toxicity Formula* (GFCH) 4. *Jade Shining* (ETHP)
Wind fire with qi deficiency	Painful, red skin lesions, usually on the lips or mouth, that come and go with colds and flus or as sequelae to some chronic diseases, frequent colds and flus; red tongue body or tip, rapid, floating pulse	Disperse wind, eliminate heat toxin, and stabilize defensive qi	Classical Formulas: 1. *Bo He Lian Qiao Pian* 2. *Liang Ge San* Patent Medicines: 1. *Yin Qiao Shang Qing Pian* 2. *Ling Qiao Jie Du Pian*	1. *Isatis Gold + Clearing* (HC) 2. *Mountain Sophora* (ETHP) 3. *Prime Response* (Jade) 4. *Viola Clear Fire Formula* (GFCH) 5. *Initial Defense* (K'an)

HIV/AIDS

HIV and AIDS have been widely publicized throughout the general press. HIV itself is not usually fatal. The opportunistic infections that occur as a result of a compromised immune system from HIV infection are what most seriously threaten patients. Clinical experience has shown that the application of Chinese herbal formulas to tonify qi, blood, yin, and yang and to restore balance among the body's organ systems can strengthen the immune response against opportunistic infections. From the perspective of TCM, there is an important window of opportunity for treatment between the awareness of HIV-positive status and a diagnosis of full-blown AIDS.

Etiology and pathology

1. Lung heat with defensive (wei) qi deficiency
2. Blood and yin deficiency with empty heat
3. Heat toxin accumulation
4. Spleen qi deficiency or sinking
5. Liver qi stagnation and heart shen disturbance

Differentiation and treatment

Although AIDS may manifest as a cold condition in its later stages, it is initially a condition of increasing low-grade heat. When in late stages cold symptoms do appear, they tend to be mixed with heat symptoms. AIDS also presents as increasingly deficient, and this deficiency is usually mixed with heat symptoms and signs.

At an asymptomatic stage, treatment focuses on immune support by tonifying wei qi (defensive qi) and harmonizing the organ systems. At various stages of AIDS, treatment can be directed toward clearing heat, detoxification, transforming damp phlegm, and moving qi and blood, in addition to tonifying qi, blood, yin and/or yang.

U.S. formulas that can be used in all types include *Enhance* (HC), *Move Mountains* (CMS), *Jade Screen* (ETHP), *Astragalus and Ligusticum Formula* (GFCH), and *IM-401* (Pro).

Type	Manifestations	Treatment Principle	Chinese Formula	U.S. Formula and Manufacturer
Lung heat with defensive qi deficiency	Fatigue, high- or low-grade fever, dry cough, dry throat, dry and hot nose, shortness of breath, recurrent sore throat, enlarged lymph nodes, neuropathy; tongue body is often red with thick dry coating or tongue has red tip and sides, pulse variable, but usually slightly rapid	Clear lung heat, consolidate defensive qi	Classical Formulas: 1. *Yu Ping Feng San* + *Yin Qiao san and Sang Ju Yin* 2. *Bu Fei Tang* + *Hao Qin Qing Dan Tang*	1. *Enhance* + *Astra Isatis* (HC) 2. *Enhance* + *Clear Heat* (HC) 3. *Strengthen Lung* + *Purge Heat* (CMS) 4. *Resilience* (CMS) + *Prime Response* (Jade) 5. *Jade Screen* + *B. Plus* (ETHP) 6. *IM-401* + *CO-197* (Pro)

Type	Manifestations	Treatment Principle	Chinese Formula	U.S. Formula and Manufacturer
Blood and yin deficiency with empty heat	Low-grade fever, insomnia, night sweats, dry skin and hair, red itchy skin or rashes, withering flesh, weight loss, dry mouth, thirst, flushed face, hot palms and soles, irritability; red tongue body with purple/blue dots or patches, scant coating or mirror tongue, rapid and thin and deep pulse	Nourish blood and yin, clear empty heat	Classical Formulas: 1. *Qing Ying Tang* 2. *Xi Jiao Di Huang Tang* 3. *Lian Xue San* 4. *Zhi Bai Di Huang Wan* 5. *Ling Jiao Gou Teng Tang*	1. *Tremella and American Ginseng* + *Clear Heat* (HC) 2. *Harmonize Kidney-Heart* + *Phlogisticlean* (CMS) 3. *Q.B.R.* + *A.V.B.* (ETHP) 4. *Temper Fire* (Jade and K'an) 5. *Nourish the Root* (TTT)
Heat toxin accumulation	Hot, red swollen gums or painful, bleeding gums, swollen lymph nodes, halitosis, constipation, red eyes, rashes, masses or tumors that come and go, frequent urinary tract infections, vaginal infections, genital skin eruptions with pain and itching, painful vesicles, facial flushing, oral sores; red or deep red tongue body with dry sticky yellow coating (or green, brown, or black coating), rapid and wiry or rapid and flooding pulse	Clear heat and detoxify	Classical Formulas: 1. *Long Dan Xie Gan Tang* 2. *Qing Wei San* 3. *Yin Chen Hao Tang* 4. *Wu Ling San* 5. *Xie Xin Tang* 6. *Zhi Bai Di Huang Wan* 7. *Huang Lian Jie Du Tang* 8. *Qing Wen Bai Du Yin* 9. *Pu Ji Xiao Du Yin* 10. *Gan Lu Xiao Du Dan*	1. *Phellostatin* + *Coptis Purge Fire Formula* (HC) 2. *Akebia Moist Heat Formula* + *Clear Heat* (HC) 3. *A.V.A.* + *Q.B.S.* (ETHP) 4. *Purge Damp Heat* + *Purge Heat* (CMS) 5. *Quell Fire* (Jade and K'an) 6. *LD-477* (Pro) 7. *Rehmannia and Scrophularia Formula* + *Coptis Relieve Toxicity Formula* (GFCH)

Type	Manifestations	Treatment Principle	Chinese Formula	U.S. Formula and Manufacturer
Spleen qi deficiency or sinking	Fatigue, heavy, lethargic feeling, anorexia, poor digestion, nausea, diarrhea, parasitic diarrhea, weight loss or wasting syndrome, yeast and fungal infections; pale flabby tongue body with white coating, soft, weak pulse	Raise spleen qi, stop diarrhea	Classical Formulas: 1. *Bu Zhong Yi Qi Tang* 2. *Li Zhong Tang* 3. *Shen Ling Bai Zhu San* 4. *Zhen Ren Yang Zang Tang* 5. *Wu Mei Wan* 6. *Huang Qi Jian Zhong Tang* 7. *Lian Li Tang*	1. *Source Qi + Six Gentlemen* (HC) 2. *Energy K + SLB* (ETHP) 3. *Wu Mei Wan Plus* (ETHP) 4. *Soothe the Center* (TTT) 5. *Prosperous Farmer* (Jade and K'an) 6. *Astragalus Formula + Ginseng and Astragalus Formula* (GFCH) 7. *Tonify Qi* (CMS)
Liver qi stagnation/heart shen disturbance	Anxiety or depression aggravated by fatigue, mood worsens as day progresses into afternoon and evening, mood swings, dream-disturbed sleep, insomnia, poor memory, palpitations, inability to concentrate; normal or slightly purple tongue with greasy white or yellow coating, wiry pulse	Move liver qi, calm spirit	Classical Formulas: 1. *Xiao Yao San* 2. *Dan Zhi Xiao Yao San* 3. *Tian Wang Bu Xin Dan* 4. *Suan Zao Ren Tang* 5. *Bai Zi Yang Xin Wan* 6. *An Shen Ding Zhi Wan* 7. *Gan Mai Da Zao Tang* Patent Medicines: 1. *Xiao Yao Wan* 2. *Shu Gan Wan* 3. *Tian Wang Bu Xin Dang* 4. *Suan Zao Ren Tang Wan* 5. *Bai Zi Yang Xin Wan* 6. *An Shen Bu Xin Wan*	1. *Ease Plus + Bupleurum Entangled Formula* (HC) 2. *Calm Dragon* (K'an) 3. *Shu Xie Tea* (ETHP) 4. *Free and Easy Wanderer Plus* (GFCH) 5. *Relaxed Wanderer + Compassionate Sage* (Jade K'an) 6. *Freeing the Moon* (TTT) 7. *RE-699* (Pro) 8. *Ease Strain + Strengthen Heart* (CMS) 9. *Comfort Shen* (CMS) 10. *Calm Spirit + Nourish Heart* (FE)

Hypertension

Hypertension is chronically high blood pressure that, in repeated tests, measures 140 or higher for systolic and 90 or higher for diastolic pressure. In TCM, hypertension is caused by an imbalance of yin and yang in the kidney and liver or by an accumulation of dampness and phlegm. It is characterized most often by headaches and dizziness, but can also manifest with symptoms of tinnitus, insomnia, palpitations, poor memory, red eyes, flushed face, and short temper, and can lead to stroke. Hypertension has historically been treated in TCM by checking the imbalance between the yin and yang, thereby preventing stroke.

Etiology and pathology

In TCM, hypertension is usually rooted in kidney and/or liver yin deficiency. This leads to liver yang rising. Thus, it is seen as an excess above and deficiency below.

1. Liver yang/fire rising disturbing the clear yang
2. Damp phlegm accumulation in the middle jiao
3. Liver yang excess with yin deficiency
4. Internal wind

Differentiation and treatment

Treatment is mainly directed toward nourishing kidney and liver yin and inducing the yang downward. U.S. formulas that can be used in all types are *Quiet Contemplative* (Jade and K'an) and *Nourish the Root* (TTT).

TType	Manifestations	Treatment Principle	Chinese Formula	U.S. Formula and Manufacturer
Liver yang/ fire rising	Dizziness, headaches, flushed face, red eyes, bitter taste in the mouth, irritability, constipation, scanty dark urine; red tongue body with yellow coating, wiry, rapid pulse	Drain liver yang/ heat, cleanse liver fire	Classical Formulas: 1. *Long Dan Xie Gan Tang* Patent Medicines: 1. *Long Dan Xie Gan Wan*	1. *Coptis Purge Fire Formula* + *Ease Plus* (HC) 2. *Drain Fire* (TTT) 3. *Quell Fire* (Jade and K'an) 4. *R.D.Y.* + *Gentiana Compound* (ETHP) 5. *LD-477* (Pro) 6. *Gentiana Drain Fire Formula* (GFCH) 7. *Purge Damp Heat* (CMS)

Type	Manifestations	Treatment Principle	Chinese Formula	U.S. Formula and Manufacturer
Damp phlegm	Heavy feeling in the head, headache, feeling of chest congestion, palpitations, nausea, vomiting, heavy and numb limbs; white greasy tongue coating, slippery pulse	Transform and eliminate damp phlegm	Classical Formulas: 1. *Ban Xia Bai Zhu Tian Ma Tang* Patent Medicines: 1. *Tian Ma Tou Tong Wan* 2. *Qing Qi Hua Tan Wan*	1. *Clear Yang* (TTT) 2. *Pinellia Phlegm Dispersing Formula* (K'an) 3. *Purge Phlegm* (CMS) 4. *HB-345* (Pro)
Liver yang excess with yin deficiency	Dizziness, headache, blurred vision, tinnitus, weak and achy low back and knees, poor memory, insomnia, palpitations, heat sensations in palms and soles; red tongue body with thin coating; thin and wiry or thin, wiry, and rapid pulse	Nourish yin and induce yang downward	Classical Formulas: 1. *Qi Ju Di Huang Wan* Patent Medicines: 1. *Qi Ju Di Huang Wan* 2. *Du Zhong Pian*	1. *Peaceful Sunset* (TTT) 2. *Bend Bamboo* (TTT) 3. *Wolfberry Compound* + *Luo Bu Ma Compound* (ETHP)
Liver wind	Severe dizziness and headaches, fainting, tremors and twitches, flushed face, aphasia, convulsion, stroke; trembling tongue or red tongue body with dry yellow or scanty coating, faint rapid pulse	Extinguish wind	Classical Formulas: 1. *Tian Ma Gou Teng Yin* 2. *Ling Jiao Gou Teng Tang* 3. *Zhen Gan Xi Feng Tang* 4. *Da Ding Feng Zhu*	1. *Gastrodia Relieve Wind* (HC) 2. *Gastrodia and Uncaria Formula* (GFCH) 3. *Purge Internal Wind* (CMS) 4. *G. Plus* (ETHP)

Hyperthyroidism

Hyperthyroidism is excessive activity of the thyroid gland. It occurs predominantly in adult females, with the highest incidence occurring between the ages of thirty and fifty. It is characterized by increased metabolism, weight loss, insomnia, palpitations, sweating, aversion to heat, tremors, and in patients with Graves disease (a condition often accompanying hyperthyroidism), an enlarged thyroid gland and bulging eyes (exophthalmia). Often, strong emotional fluctuations accompany hyperthyroidism. TCM attributes hyperthyroidism to phlegm fire obstructing the meridians of the neck and excessive emotional stimulation.

Etiology and pathology

Qi stagnation is the main cause. The liver, kidney, heart, and spleen are the main organs involved.

1. At initial stages, hyperthyroidism manifests as an excess condition: liver qi stagnation with liver fire rising, phlegm obstruction, and blood stagnation.
2. At later or chronic stages, a deficient condition manifests as liver, kidney, and heart yin deficiency with spleen qi deficiency.
3. At the severe stage in an acute attack, a critical combination of excess and deficiency occurs: liver and kidney yin deficiency with liver yang rising, internal wind, and possible yin exhaustion with yang collapse.

Differentiation and treatment

There are usually three types. Treatment for the excess condition is directed toward spreading and moving liver qi, draining fire, and transforming phlegm. For the deficient condition, yin is nourished and spleen qi tonified. In the acute stage, internal wind is extinguished. U.S. formulas that can be used in all types are *Adrenosen* (HC) and *Q.B.H.* (ETHP).

Type	Manifestations	Treatment Principle	Chinese Formula	U.S. Formula and Manufacturer
Qi stagnation with phlegm obstruction	Enlarged, but soft and painless thyroid, hypochondriac distension and pain, frequent sighing; thin, greasy tongue coating, wiry, slippery pulse	Spread and move liver qi, transform and eliminate phlegm	Classical Formulas: 1. *Si Hai Shu Yu Wan* + *Hai Zao Yu Hu Tang* Patent Medicines: 1. *Hai Zao Wan*	1. *Pinellia Phlegm Dispersing Formula* (K'an) 2. *Bupleurum D Formula* (GFCH) 3. *Cluster Dissolving* (CMS)

Type	Manifestations	Treatment Principle	Chinese Formula	U.S. Formula and Manufacturer
Liver fire	Enlarged thyroid, exophthalmia, irritability, flushed face, aversion to heat, sweating, bitter taste in mouth, red eyes; thin yellow tongue coating, red tongue body, rapid, wiry pulse	Clear heat, drain fire	Classical Formulas: 1. *Long Dan Xie Gan Tang* + *Zao Yao San* 2. *Dan Zhi Xiao Yao San* Patent Medicines: 1. *Long Dan Xie Gan Wan*	1. *Coptis Purge Fire* (HC) 2. *Drain Fire* + *Smooth Passage* (TTT) 3. *Quell Fire* (Jade and K'an) + *Pinellia Phlegm Dispersing Formula* (K'an) 4. *R.D.Y.* + *Green Xiao Yao San* (ETHP) 5. *Detox Compound* (CHC) 6. *LD-477* (Pro) 7. *Gentiana Drain Fire Formula* (GFCH) 8. *Purge Damp Heat* (CMS)
Heart and liver yin deficiency	Palpitations, irritability, insomnia, dream-disturbed sleep, hypochondriac pain, dry mouth, no significant thyroid enlargement; red tongue, rapid, wiry pulse	Nourish heart and liver yin, calm spirit	Classical Formulas: 1. *Tian Wang Bu Xin Dan* + *Yi Guan Jian* Patent Medicines: 1. *Tian Wang Bu Xin Wan* 2. *An Shen Bu Xin Wan* 3. *Ming Mu Di Huang Wan*	1. *Heavenly Emperor's Formula* (GFCH) 2. *Ming Mu Formula* (GFCH) 3. *Calm Spirit* + *Schizandra Dreams* (HC) 4. *Fertile Garden* (HC) 5. *Energy S* (ETHP) 6. *Strengthen Liver* + *Strengthen Heart* (CMS) 7. *Clear the Soul* + *Root the Spirit* (TTT)

Hypochondriac Pain

Hypochondriac pain, a common complaint in the clinical setting, refers to a pain felt on one or both sides of the hypochondrium. It is included in liver disease, biliary disorders, and intercostal neuralgia in Western medicine.

Etiology and pathology

The liver is the main organ involved in hypochondriac pain.

1. Liver qi stagnation
2. Liver blood stagnation
3. Liver and gallbladder damp heat
4. Liver yin deficiency

Differentiation and treatment

U.S. formulas that can be used in all types include *Break Into a Smile* (TTT).

Type	Manifestations	Treatment Principle	Chinese Formula	U.S. Formula and Manufacturer
Liver qi stagnation	Distention and wandering pain in the hypochondriac region aggravated by emotional stress, accompanied by full sensation in the chest, poor appetite, frequent belching, irritability, poor sleep; thin white tongue coating, wiry pulse	Soothe the liver, regulate qi circulation, and stop pain	Classical Formulas: 1. *Si Ni San* 2. *Chai Hu Shu Gan San* Patent Medicines: 1.*Chai Hu Shu Gan Wan*	1. *Break Into a Smile* (TTT) 2. *Chai Hu Shu Gan San Plus* (ETHP)
Liver blood stasis	Localized sharp pain aggravated at night, pain worse with pressure, possible hypochondriac mass; dark purplish tongue body and deep choppy pulse	Circulate qi and blood, remove blood stasis, and stop pain	Classical Formulas: 1. *Xue Fu Zhu Yu Tang* Patent Medicines: 1. *Xue Fu Zhu Yu Tang Wan*	1. *Disperse Blood* (CMS) 2. *Tang Kuei and Salvia Formula* (GFCH) 3. *Q.B.A.* (ETHP)

Type	Manifestations	Treatment Principle	Chinese Formula	U.S. Formula and Manufacturer
Liver and gallbladder damp heat	Stabbing pain with burning sensation particularly in the right hypochondriac region, accompanied by chills and fever, bitter taste, irritability, nausea and vomiting, red or inflamed eyes, scanty urine; red tongue body with yellow coating, wiry rapid pulse	Clear heat, resolve dampness, soothe the liver, and promote the function of the gallbladder	Classical Formulas: 1. *Long Dan Xie Gan Tang* Patent Medicines: 1. *Long Dan Xie Gan Wan*	1. *Quell Fire* (K'an and Jade) 2. *Gentiana Drain Fire Formula* (GFCH) 3. *Coptis Purge Fire Formula* (HC)
Liver yin deficiency	Lingering, dull pain in both hypochondriac regions, dry mouth, restlessness, blurred vision, dizziness, afternoon fever, spontaneous sweating; red tongue body with scanty coating, thin rapid pulse	Nourish liver yin and relieve pain	Classical Formulas: 1. *Yi Guan Jian*	1. *Strengthen Liver* (CMS) 2. *Radio-Support* (TTT)

Hypomenorrhea

Hypomenorrhea refers to the condition in which the menstrual cycle is essentially normal except that the menstrual flow is noticeably reduced to a few drops; or, the cycle lasts less than two days and the flow is scanty.

Etiology and pathology

1. Blood deficiency
2. Kidney deficiency
3. Blood stagnation
4. Phlegm damp

Differentiation and treatment

U.S. formulas that can be used in all types include *Precious Sea* (WT).

Type	Manifestations	Treatment Principle	Chinese Formula	U.S. Formula and Manufacturer
Blood deficiency	Scanty, light-colored menses, dizziness, blurred vision, palpitations, sallow complexion, pale lips; pale tongue body, white coating, thin and weak pulse	Tonify the blood and regulate menstruation	Classical Formulas: 1. *Ba Zhen Tang* Patent Medicines: 1. *Ba Zhen Yi Mu Wan* 2. *Nu Zhi Bao*	1. *Precious Sea* (WT) 2. *Women's Precious* (Jade and K'an) 3. *Eight Treasures* (HC) 4. *Tonify Blood* (CMS)
Kidney deficiency	Thin, scanty menses, light or dark red menses, soreness and weakness of the low back and knees, pain in the heel, dizziness, tinnitus, cold feeling in the lower abdomen, nocturia; pale tongue body, deep and weak pulse	Tonify the kidney and regulate menstruation	Classical Formulas: 1. *Gui Shen Wan* 2. *Zuo Gui Wan* (more kidney yin deficiency) 3. *You Gui Wan* (more kidney yang deficiency) 4. *Nu Bao*	1. *Unicorn Pearl* (WT) *Note:* For kidney yin deficiency, add *Ease Journey-Yin* (WT). For kidney yang deficiency, add *Ease Journey-Yang* (WT)
Blood stasis	Scanty, dark purple menses with clots, distending pain in the lower abdomen aggravated by pressure and alleviated after discharge of clots; normal or dark red tongue body, or a tongue with fine purple spots, thready and uneven, or wiry and uneven pulse	Circulate blood, remove blood stasis, and regulate menstruation	Classical Formulas: 1. *Tao Hong Si Wu Tang* Patent Medicines: 1. *Gui Zhi Fu Ling Wan*	1. *Women's Rhythm* (K'an and Jade) 2. *Women's Chamber* (K'an and Jade) *Note:* For blood stasis with cold stagnation, combine with *Women's Journey* (Jade and K'an) or *Warm the Menses* (WT)
Phlegm damp	Scanty, sticky, light-colored menses, obesity, full sensation in the chest, nausea, profuse sticky leukorrhea; pale tongue body, white greasy coating, slippery pulse	Eliminate damp, resolve phlegm, and regulate menstruation	Classical Formulas: 1. *Cang Fu Dao Tan Wan* Patent Medicines: 1. *Cang Fu Dao Tan Wan*	1. *Clear the Palace* (WT) 2. *Lucid Channel* (K'an) 3. *Lucid Clarity* (Jade) 4. *Disperse Moisture* (CMS)

Impotence

Impotence refers to the inability to achieve or maintain an erect penis, resulting in the inability to engage in normal sexual activity.

Etiology and pathology

1. Excessive sexual activity, masturbation, and so forth, leading to kidney deficiency
2. Fear, fright, and worry, leading to qi stagnation or shen disturbance
3. Internal damp heat retention

Differentiation and treatment

U.S. formulas that can be used in all types include *Strengthen the Root* (TTT) and *Nine Flavor Tea* (HC).

Type	Manifestations	Treatment Principle	Chinese Formula	U.S. Formula and Manufacturer
Kidney deficiency	Poor erection of penis or erection that lasts only for seconds, pale complexion, cold limbs, dizziness, blurred vision, poor spirit, soreness in the lumbar region and knee joints, frequent urination; pale tongue body with white coating; deep, thready pulse palpitations and insomnia in some cases	Reinforce kidney yang and warm the lower jiao	Classical Formulas: 1. *Wu Zi Yan Zong Wan* Patent Medicines: 1. *Nan Bao* 2. *Sea Horse Tonic Pill* 3. *Tze Pao San Pian Wan*	1. *MA-511* (Pro) 2. *TCB4 Eucommia Combination* (MG) 3. *Essential Yang Formula* (GFCH) 4. *Tian Kui T-M* (ETHP)
Impairment of heart and spleen	Poor erection of penis, fatigue, poor sleep, pale complexion; pale tongue body, thin and greasy coating, thready pulse	Tonify the heart and spleen	Classical Formulas: 1. *Gui Pi Tang* Patent Medicines: 1. *Gui Pi Wan*	1. *Gather Vitality* (K'an and Jade) 2. *Ginseng Nourishing Formula* (GFCH) 3. *General Tonic Formula* (GFCH)

Type	Manifestations	Treatment Principle	Chinese Formula	U.S. Formula and Manufacturer
Downward flowing of damp heat	Inability to achieve erection, wet scrotum with foul smell, bitter taste in the mouth, thirst, scanty urine, soreness in the lower limbs; greasy tongue coating, rapid soft pulse	Eliminate damp heat	Classical Formulas: 1. *Long Dan Xie Gan Tang* 2. *Zhi Bai Di Huang Wan* Patent Medicines 1. *Long Dan Xie Gan Wan* 2. *Zhi Bai Di Huang Wan*	1. *Quell Fire* (K'an and Jade) 2. *Temper Fire* (K'an and Jade) 3. *Clear the Root* (TTT) 4. *Gentiana Compound* (ETHP) 5. *Gentiana Drain Fire Formula* (GFCH)

Infantile Cough

Cough is a common clinical symptom, mainly present in respiratory illness. It may occur at any time of the year but occurs usually in winter and spring. In children, cough may be classified into two types: external and internal. The former is more common.

Etiology and pathology

1. Cough caused by exogenous pathogenic factors
   - Wind cold
   - Wind heat
2. Stagnation of phlegm in the interior
   - Phlegm damp
   - Phlegm heat
3. Weak constitution
   - Yin deficiency
   - Lung qi deficiency

Differentiation and treatment

U.S. formulas that can be used in all types include *Yin Chao Junior* (HC) and *Children's Herbal Sentinal* (TTT).

Type	Manifestations	Treatment Principle	Chinese Formula	U.S. Formula and Manufacturer
Wind cold	Recurrent heavy cough, itchiness in the throat, thin white sputum, chills, fever, stuffy nose with watery discharge, headache and general bodily achiness (pantalgia); thin white tongue coating, floating, tense pulse	Disperse wind cold, circulate lung qi to stop the cough	Classical Formulas: 1. *Jin Fu Cao San* Patent Medicines: 1. *Ma Hsing Zhi Ke Pian*	1. *Prime Rescue* (Jade) + *AS-135* (Pro)
Wind heat	Cough with yellowish sputum that is difficult to expectorate, thirst, red, painful, swollen throat, fever with aversion to wind, slight sweating, turbid nasal discharge; red tongue tip with thin, slightly yellow coating, floating and rapid pulse	Disperse wind, clear heat, circulate lung qi and resolve the phlegm	Classical Formulas: 1. *Sang Ju Yin* Patent Medicines: 1. *San She Dan Chuan Bei Ye* 2. *She Dan Chuan Bei Ye*	1. *Prime Response* (Jade) 2. *Initial Defense* (K'an) *Note:* For severe cases, add *Clear Air* (HC) or *AS-137* (Pro).
Phlegm heat	Cough with abundant thick yellow sputum, fever, flushed face, red lips, thirst, restlessness, epistaxis (nosebleed), dry stool, dark urine; red tongue body with yellow, greasy coating, slippery and rapid pulse	Clear the lung heat and resolve phlegm	Classical Formulas: 1. *Qin Jin Hua Tan Tang* Patent Medicines: 1. *San She Dan Chuan Bei Ye* 2. *Qing Qi Hua Tan Wan*	1. *AS-137* (Pro) 2. *Clear Air* (HC) 3. *Chest Relief* (CMS)
Phlegm dampness	Cough with thin, white, and productive sputum, loss of appetite, fullness of the chest, listlessness, pale complexion; pale tongue body, white, greasy coating, slippery pulse	Invigorate the spleen to dry the dampness, and resolve phlegm to relieve cough	Classical Formulas: 1. *Er Chen Tang* Patent Medicines: 1. *Er Chen Wan* 2. *Chuan Bei Pi Pa* syrup (for chronic cough)	1. *Lucid Channal* (K'an) 2. *Lucid Clarity* (Jade) *Note:* For spleen deficiency symptoms, add *Prosperous Farmer* (K'an and Jade).

Type	Manifestations	Treatment Principle	Chinese Formula	U.S. Formula and Manufacturer
Yin deficiency	Dry cough, or cough with scanty thick sputum that is difficult to expectorate, blood-tinged sputum, dryness in the mouth and throat, flushed cheeks, tidal fever, night sweats, feverish sensation in the palms and soles; red tongue body with scanty coating, thin and rapid pulse	Nourish yin, moisten dryness, clear the lung, and stop cough	Classical Formulas: 1. *Sha Shen Mai Dong Tang* 2. *Bai He Gu Jin Tang* 3. *Chuan Bei Pi Pa Ye*	1. *Wise Judge* (K'an and Jade) 2. *Lily Preserve Metal Formula* (GFCH)
Lung qi deficiency	Weak cough with thin and clear or white sputum, pale complexion, shortness of breath, aversion to speaking, low voice, profuse sweating; pale and tender tongue body, thin and weak pulse	Tonify the lung and spleen qi	Classical Formulas: 1. *Liu Jun Zi Tang* Patent Medicines 1. *Li Fei*	1. *Six Gentlemen Formula* (GFCH) 2. *Prosperous Farmer* (K'an and Jade) 3. *Ginseng and Gecko Herbal Formula* (HC)

Infantile Diarrhea

Infantile diarrhea is characterized by frequent defecation and loose or watery stools. It is one of the most common diseases in children. The younger the child, the higher the morbidity. It is mostly seen in children under the age of two.

Etiology and pathology

1. Improper feeding, overfeeding
2. Invasion of exopathogens
   - Cold damp
   - Damp heat
3. Weakness of spleen and stomach
4. Spleen and kidney yang deficiency

Differentiation and treatment

U.S. formulas that can be used in all types include *Children's Herbal Sentinel* (TTT).

Type	Manifestations	Treatment Principle	Chinese Formula	U.S. Formula and Manufacturer
Overfeeding	Abdominal distention and pain, followed by diarrhea and relieved by defecation; sour and foul-smelling or rotten egg–smelling stools and intestinal gas, belching with fetid gas, vomiting; thick greasy or curdy tongue coating	Promote and regulate the stomach to arrest diarrhea	Classical Formulas: 1. *Bao He Wan* 2. *Da Shan Zha Wan*	1. *Meal Mover* (CMS) 2. *Quiet Digestion* (HC) 3. *Purge Qi* (CMS)
Cold damp	Watery stool with foam and little foul smell, bowel sounds, abdominal pain, chills and fever, watery nasal discharge; thin, white, moist tongue coating	Warm the middle jiao, dispel cold, and resolve damp to arrest diarrhea	Classical Formulas: 1. *Huo Xiang Zheng Qi San* 2. *Wei Ling Tang* Patent Medicines: 1. *Huo Xiang Zheng Qi Shui* 2. *Huo Xiang Zheng Qi Wan*	1. *Prime Relief* (Jade) 2. *Early Comfort* (K'an) 3. *Ease Digestion Formula* (GFCH) *Note:* For watery diarrhea, add *Water Way* (K'an).
Damp heat	Dark-yellow stool with strong smell or with a little mucous or spotted stools, redness and burning sensation in the anus, scanty dark urine; red tongue body, yellow and greasy coating	Clear damp heat to arrest diarrhea	Classical Formulas: 1. *Ge Gen Qin Lian Tang* Patent Medicines: 1. *Huang Lian Su Pian* 2. *Xiang Lian Wan*	1. *Copticlear* (K'an) 2. *Phellostatin* (HC)
Spleen deficiency	Loose stools immediately after feeding with little smell and with white milk masses or undigested food, sallow complexion, half-closed eyes when sleeping, listlessness; pale tongue body, thin white tongue coating	Invigorate the spleen and replenish qi	Classical Formulas: 1. *Shen Ling Bai Zhu San* Patent Medicines: 1. *Shen Ling Bai Zhu Wan*	1. *Source Qi* (HC) 2. *Prosperious Farmer* (Jade and K'an) 3. *Arouse Vigor* (Jade and K'an)
Spleen and kidney yang deficiency	Diarrhea that has become chronic, discharge of stools immediately after feeding, indigestion, cold limbs, intolerance of cold, emaciation; pale tongue body, white tongue coating	Tonify the spleen and warm the kidney	Classical Formulas: 1. *Fu Zi Li Zhong Wan* 2. *Si Shen Wan* Patent Medicines: 1. *Si Shen Wan* 2. *Fu Zi Li Zhong Wan*	1. *Purge Cold* (CMS) + *Consolidate Qi* (CMS)

Infertility

If a woman is unable to become pregnant for more than two years after trying on a regular basis, and the reproductive function of her male sexual partner is normal, the condition is referred to as primary infertility. If a woman fails to become pregnant again for more than two years after a previous labor or miscarriage, the condition is termed secondary infertility.

Etiology and pathology

1. Kidney deficiency
   - Kidney yang deficiency
   - Kidney yin deficiency
2. Liver qi stagnation
3. Phlegm damp
4. Blood stagnation

Differentiation and treatment

U.S. formulas that can be used in all types include *Planting Seeds* (WT) and *Maternal Herbal* (HC).

Type	Manifestations	Treatment Principle	Chinese Formula	U.S. Formula and Manufacturer
Kidney yang deficiency	Infertility, prolonged menstrual cycle with scanty and light-colored flow or ammenorrhea, dark complexion, soreness and weakness of the loins and knees, low sex drive, clear and profuse urine, loose stool; pale tongue body, white coating, deep thin pulse, or deep slow pulse	Tonify kidney yang, disperse cold, and warm the uterus	Classical Formulas: 1. *Yu Ling Zhu* 2. *Si Wu Tang* 3. *Si Jun Zi Tang* Patent Medicines: 1. *Ai Fu Nuan Gong Wan*	1. *Unicorn Pearl* (WT) 2. *Warm the Mansion* (WT)

Type	Manifestations	Treatment Principle	Chinese Formula	U.S. Formula and Manufacturer
Kidney yin deficiency	Infertility, shortened menstrual cycle with scanty red flow and absence of clots, or normal menstruation with other symptoms and signs including emaciation, soreness, and weakness of the lumbar region and knees, dizziness, blurred vision, palpitations, insomnia, irritability, dry mouth, heat sensation in the palms, soles, and chest, afternoon low-grade fever; red tongue with scanty coating, thready, rapid pulse	Tonify kidney yin and regulate the Chong and Ren channels	Classical Formulas: 1. *Yang Jing Zhong Yu Tang* + *Er Zhi Wan* 2. *Zuo Gui Wan*	1. *Growing Jade* (WT) *Note:* To strengthen the action of tonifying kidney yin, add *Ease Journey-Yin* (WT). With yin deficiency with deficient heat, use together with *Temper Fire* (Jade and K'an).
Liver qi stagnation	Infertility, irregular menstrual cycle with hesitant, scanty, and dark flow with clots, dysmenorrhea, premenstrual distending pain in the breasts, mental depression, irritability, normal or dark red tongue body, thin and white coating, wiry pulse	Circulate the liver qi and regulate Chong and Ren channels	Classical Formulas: 1. *Kai Yu Zhong Yu Tang* 2. *Xiao Yao San* Patent Medicines: 1. *Xiao Yao Wan* 2. *Shu Gan Wan*	1. *Relaxed Wanderer* (K'an and Jade) 2. *Woman's Balance* (HC) 3. *Freeing the Moon* (WT) 4. *Bupleurum and Tang Kuei Formula* (GFCH) *Note:* For heat transformation of liver qi, add *Free Flow* (WT).
Phlegm damp	Infertility, overweight constitution, prolonged menstrual cycle or ammenorrhea, profuse, sticky vaginal discharge, pale complexion, dizziness, palpitations, feeling of suffocation, nausea; white, sticky tongue coating, slippery pulse	Resolve phlegm and eliminate damp	Classical Formulas: 1. *Qi Gong Wan* + *Shi cang pu* Patent Medicines: 1. *Er Chen Wan*	1. *Clear the Palace* (WT) 2. *Lucid Channel* (K'an) 3. *Lucid Clarity* (Jade)

Type	Manifestations	Treatment Principle	Chinese Formula	U.S. Formula and Manufacturer
Blood stagnation	Infertility, prolonged menstrual cycle with scanty and dark-purplish flow with clots, dysmenorrhea aggravated by pressure; dark-purplish tongue body or purple spots on the border of the tongue, thready, wiry pulse	Promote blood circulation and remove blood stasis	Classical Formulas: 1. *Shao Fu Zhu Yu Tang*	1. *Women's Rhythm* (Jade and K'an) 2. *Women's Chamber* (K'an) 3. *Women's Palace* (Jade) *Note:* For blood stasis with cold, add either *Women's Journey* (Jade and (K'an) or *Warm the Menses* (WT).

Insomnia

Insomnia is characterized by disturbed sleep or frequent inability to fall asleep. In mild cases, the patient has difficulty falling asleep or awakens frequently. In severe cases, the patient may not be able to fall asleep for an entire night, which, if prolonged, will lead to other pathologies.

Etiology and pathology

1. Deficiency of the heart and spleen
2. Disharmony between the heart and kidney
3. Upward attack of the liver fire
4. Dysfunction of the stomach
5. Deficiency of the heart and gallbladder

Differentiation and treatment

U.S. formulas that can be used in all types include *SL-749* (Pro).

Type	Manifestations	Treatment Principle	Chinese Formula	U.S. Formula and Manufacturer
Deficiency of the heart and spleen	Dream-disturbed sleep, easily woken up, palpitations, poor memory, dizziness, blurred vision, lassitude, listlessness, pale complexion; pale tongue body, thin white coating, thready and weak pulse	Invigorate the spleen qi, tonify the heart blood to tranquilize the mind	Classical Formulas: 1. *Gui Pi Tang* Patent Medicines: 1. *Bai Zi Yang Xin Wan* 2. *Gui Pi Wan*	1. *Gather Vitality* (Jade and K'an) 2. *Compassionate Sage: Heart Spirit* (Jade and K'an) 3. *Shen-Gem* (HC) 4. *Calm Spirit* (HC) 5. *Red Horse: Wood Create Fire* (Jade) 6. *Women's Precious* (Jade and K'an)
Disharmony between the heart and kidney	Difficulty in falling asleep with restlessness, palpitations, dizziness, nocturnal emission, burning sensation in the palms, soles, and chest, dry mouth with scanty saliva; red tongue body with little coating, thin and rapid pulse	Nourish yin, purge fire, tonify heart, and tranquilize the mind	Classical Formulas: 1. *Huang Lian E Jiao Tang* 2. *Zhu Sha An Shen Wan* Patent Medicines: 1. *Tian Wang Bu Xin Dan*	1. *Celestial Emperor's Blend* (K'an) 2. *Compassionate Sage: Heart Spirit + Temper Fire* (Jade and K'an) 3. *Quiet Contemplative: Kidney Yin* (Jade and K'an) + *Compassionate Sage* (Jade and K'an)
Upward attack of liver fire	Dream-disturbed sleep, irritability and hot temper, poor appetite, thirst, bloodshot eyes, bitter taste in the mouth, dark-yellow urine, dry stool; red tongue body, yellow coating, wiry and rapid pulse	Clear fire from the liver and heart, tranquilize the mind	Classical Formulas: 1. *Long Dan Xie Gan Tang* Patent Medicines: 1. *Long Dan Xie Gan Wan*	1. *PM-637* (Pro) 2. *Woman's Balance* (HC) 3. *Quell Fire: Liver Fire and Damp Heat* (Jade and K'an) 4. *HB-345* (Pro) 5. *New Gastrodia Relieve Wind Formula* (HC)

Type	Manifestations	Treatment Principle	Chinese Formula	U.S. Formula and Manufacturer
Dysfunction of the stomach	Insomnia, fullness and distention in the chest and stomach, aversion to food, belching, acid regurgitation, nausea, vomiting, restlessness, bitter taste in the mouth, heaviness of the head or dizziness; yellow, greasy tongue coating, slippery and rapid pulse	Promote digestion to remove undigested food, clear heat and resolve phlegm	Patent Medicines: 1. *Bao He Wan*	1. *Quiet Digestion* (HC) 2. *Meal Mover* (CMS) 3. *Purge Qi* (CMS) 4. *Lucid Clarity: Transform Phlegm* (Jade) + *GI-337* (Pro) 5. *Lucid Channel* (K'an)
Gallbladder and heart qi deficiency	Dream-disturbed sleep, palpitation, shortness of breath, lassitude, profuse, clear urine; pale tongue body, thin, wiry pulse	Tonify qi and tranquilize the mind	Classical Formulas: 1. *Suan Zao Ren Tang* Patent Medicines: 1. *An Shen Ding Zhi Wan* 2. *Suan Zan Ren Tang Wan*	1. *SL-749* (Pro) 2. *Red Horse: Wood Creates Fire* (Jade)

Insufficient Lactation

Insufficient lactation refers to the clinical manifestation of insufficient breast milk to feed the baby. In some cases, there is no milk secretion at all.

Etiology and pathology

1. Constitutional spleen and stomach deficiency
2. Profuse loss of blood during delivery leading to qi and blood deficiency
3. Mental depression leading to liver qi stagnation

Differentiation and treatment

There are two types of insufficient lactation according to Chinese medicine: deficiency and excess. Treatment is directed toward tonifying and moving qi and blood. U.S. formulas that can be used in all types include *Eight Treasures* (HC) and *Precious Sea* (WT).

Type	Manifestations	Treatment Principle	Chinese Formula	U.S. Formula and Manufacturer
Qi and blood deficiency	Insufficient, or absence of, milk secretion after delivery, or scanty, light, dilute milk secretion, absence of breast distention, pale complexion, lassitude, palpitations, night sweating, spontaneous sweating, poor appetite; pale tongue body, weak, thready, or rapid pulse	Tonify qi and blood	Classical Formulas: 1. *Shi Quan Da Bu Tang* 2. *Ba Zhen Tang* Patent Medicines: 1. *Ba Zhen Wan* 2. *Shi Quan Da Bu Wan*	1. *General Tonic Formula* (GFCH) 2. *Women's Precious* (Jade and K'an)
Liver qi stagnation	Absence of milk secretion after delivery or a sudden stoppage of milk secretion during nursing as a result of emotional stimulation, distended, painful breasts, possibly developing into mastitis, hypochondriac distention, mental depression, poor appetite, frequent belching; normal or slightly flabby tongue, wiry, thready pulse	Move liver qi and tonify spleen and stomach qi	Classical Formulas: 1. *Xiao Yao San* 2. *Chai Hu Shu Gan San* Patent Medicines: 1. *Xiao Yao Wan* 2. *Shu Gan Wan*	1. *Bupleurum Entangled Qi Formula* (HC) 2. *Yellow Xiaoyao San* (ETHP) 3. *Freeing the Moon* (TTT) 4. *Free and Easy Wanderer Plus* (GFCH)

Irregular Menstruation

Irregular menstruation means that a woman's period does not occur at regular cyclic intervals. It is termed irregular if it is more than seven days early or more than seven days late.

Etiology and pathology

Imbalance between qi and blood, dysfunction of the Chong and Ren meridians, and disorder of the Sea of Blood may all be responsible for this condition. Clinically, liver qi stagnation and kidney deficiency are most commonly encountered.

1. Liver qi stagnation
2. Kidney deficiency

Differentiation and treatment

U.S. formulas that can be used in all types include *Women's Balance* (HC) and *Female Treasure* (WT).

Type	Manifestations	Treatment Principle	Chinese Formula	U.S. Formula and Manufacturer
Liver qi stagnation	Irregular menstrual cycle, with either profuse or scanty discharge of menses, clots in the flow, fullness or distending pain of the lower abdomen, chest, hypochondrium, and breast, belching, poor appetite, depression; thin and white tongue coating, wiry pulse	Soothe the liver, regulate Chong and Ren meridians	Classical Formulas: 1. *Xiao Yao San* Patent Medicines: 1. *Xiao Yao Wan* 2. *Shu Gan Wan*	1. *Relaxed Wanderer* (Jade and K'an) 2. *Woman's Balance* (HC) 3. *Bupleurum and Tang Kuei Formula* (GFCH)
Kidney deficiency	Irregular menstrual cycle, profuse or scanty pale menses, dizziness, tinnitus, soreness and weakness of the low back, and hips, hollow pain in the lower abdomen, nocturia, loose stool; pale tongue body, thin coating, deep and weak pulse	Tonify the kidney and regulate the Chong and Ren meridians	Classical Formulas: 1. *Gu Yin Jian + Rou Gui, Fu Zi, Bu Gu Zhi* Patent Medicines: 1. *Nu Ke Ba Zhen Wan* 2. *Nu Zhi Bao*	1. *Unicorn Pearl* (TTT) 2. *Astra Essence* (HC)

Late Menstrual Cycle

A menstrual period delayed seven or more days than normal is considered a late menstrual cycle.

Etiology and pathology

1. Blood cold
   - Excess cold
   - Deficient cold
2. Blood deficiency
3. Qi stagnation

Differentiation and treatment

U.S. formulas that can be used in all types include *Growing Jade* (HC).

Type	Manifestations	Treatment Principle	Chinese Formula	U.S. Formula and Manufacturer
Blood cold—excess	Delayed menstruation with scanty, dark menses mixed with clots, cold pain in the lower abdomen that can be relieved by warmth, intolerance of cold, cold extremities; white tongue coating, deep and tense pulse	Warm the channels, relieve cold	Classical Formulas: 1. *Wen Jing Tang* 2. *Gui Zhi Fu Ling Wan*	1. *Women's Journey* (Jade and K'an) 2. *Warm the Menses* (WT) *Note:* If blood stasis present, add *Women's Chamber* (K'an) or *Women's Palace* (Jade).
Blood cold—deficient	Delayed menstruation with scanty, pink-colored and watery menses, without clots, dull pain in the lower abdomen that can be decreased by pressure and warmth, soreness and weakness of the loins, profuse, clear urine, loose stool; pale tongue body, white coating, deep and slow or thready and weak pulse	Tonify yang and regulate menstruation	Classical Formulas: 1. *Ai Fu Nuan Gong Wan* Patent Medicines: 1. *Ai Fu Nuan Gong Wan*	1. *Warm the Mansion* (WT) *Note:* Above can be used together with *Warm the Palace* (WT) to strengthen the effect of tonifying kidney yang.
Blood deficiency	Delayed menstrual cycle with scanty, light-colored menses without clots, dull, hollow pain in the lower abdomen, dizziness, blurred vision, palpitations, poor sleep, pale or sallow complexion; pale tongue body, thin and feeble pulse	Tonify blood and regulate menstruation	Classical Formulas: 1. *Da Bu Yuan Jian* 2. *Ren Shen Yang Ying Tang* 3. *Gui Pi Tang* Patent Medicines: 1. *Ba Zhen Wan*	1. *Women's Precious* (Jade and K'an) 2. *Eight Treasures* (HC) 3. *Ginseng Nourishing Formula* (GFCH) 4. *Gather Vitality* (Jade and K'an)
Qi stagnation	Delayed menstrual cycle, scanty, dark menses mixed with clots, distention in the lower abdomen, distending pain in the chest, abdomen, hypochondrium, and breasts; wiry pulse	Circulate qi and regulate menstruation	Classical Formulas: 1. *Xiao Yao San* Patent Medicines: 1. *Xiao Yao Wan* 2. *Shu Gan Wan*	1. *Relaxed Wanderer* (Jade and K'an) 2. *Bupleurum and Tang Kuei Formula* (GFCH)

Leukorrhea

Leukorrhea is a condition of persistent and excessive vaginal discharge with abnormal color, quality, and odor. In Western medicine, this condition may be caused by vaginitis, cervicitis, endometritis, tumor, or weakness of the body constitution.

Etiology and pathology

The spleen and kidney are the primary organs involved in leukorrhea.

1. Spleen injury resulting from improper diet, overstrain, and stress
2. Kidney deficiency from excessive sexual activity or multiple childbirths
3. Invasion by damp which turns to damp heat

Differentiation and treatment

U.S. formulas that can be used in all types include *Isatis Cooling Formula* (HC).

Type	Manifestations	Treatment Principle	Chinese Formula	U.S. Formula and Manufacturer
Spleen deficiency	Persistent white or yellowish sticky leukorrhea without foul smell, sallow complexion, general lassitude, anorexia, loose stool; pale tongue body with white sticky coating, moderate, weak pulse	Reinforce spleen qi, resolve dampness, and resolve leukorrhea	Classical Formulas: 1. *Wan Dai Tang* 2. *Shen Ling Bai Zhu San*	1. *Golden Rose* (ETHP) 2. *Clear Palace* (WT) 3. *Six Gentlemen* (HC)
Kidney deficiency	Copious thin white vaginal discharge, soreness in the lower back, loose stool, cold sensation in the lower abdomen, frequent and excessive urination; pale tongue body with white coating, deep, slow pulse	Warm and tonify kidney qi, consolidate Ren and Dai meridians, and stop discharge	Classical Formulas: 1. *Nei Bu Wan* Patent Medicines: 1. *Ji Sheng Shen Qi Wan*	1. *Harmonize Spleen and Kidney* + *Consolidate Qi* (CMS)
Damp heat (toxic damp) retention	Copious, foul-smelling yellowish vaginal discharge, purulent, itching, sinking pain in the lower abdomen, bitter taste in the mouth, thirst, dry stool, scanty urination; sticky yellow tongue coating, rapid, slippery pulse	Clear heat, resolve damp, and stop leukorrhea	Classical Formulas: 1. *Long Dan Xie Gan Tang* 2. *Zhi Bai Di Huang Wan* Patent Medicines: 1. *Long Dan Xie Gan Wan* 2. *Chien Chin Chih Tai Wan* 3. *Yu Dai Wan*	1. *Quell Fire* (K'an and Jade) 2. *Drain the Jade Valley* (WT) 3. *Temper Fire* (K'an and Jade) 4. *Purge Damp Heat* (CMS)

Lumbar Pain

Lumbar pain refers to unilateral, bilateral, or centrally located pain along the spinal column in the lumbar region. In TCM, it is closely associated with kidney disorder, for the lumbar region is the residence of the kidneys.

Etiology and pathology

1. Invasion by pathogenic damp cold
2. Invasion by pathogenic damp heat
3. Trauma due to sprain or contusion
4. Kidney deficiency

Differentiation and treatment

U.S. formulas that can be used in all types include *PA-623* (Pro) and *Rehmannia 8* (HC).

Type	Manifestations	Treatment Principle	Chinese Formula	U.S. Formula and Manufacturer
Damp cold	Low back pain usually occurring after exposure to cold and damp and aggravated on rainy days, cold and heavy sensation and stiffness of the muscles in the dorsolumbar region, limitation of extension and flexion of the back; white and greasy tongue coating, deep, moderate pulse, or deep slow pulse	Expel damp cold, warm channels to relieve pain	Classical Formulas: 1. *Gan Jiang Ling Zhu Tang*	1. *AR-125* (Pro) 2. *Mobility 2* (HC) 3. *Meridian Circulation* (Jade)
Damp heat	Pain with hot, burning sensation in lumbar areas especially on warm, humid days, yellow urine; red tongue body, yellow and greasy coating, rapid, soft pulse	Clear heat and resolve damp, dredge the channels and collaterals to stop pain	Classical Formulas: 1. *Jia Wei Er Miao San* 2. *Qi Wei Cang Bai San* Patent Medicines: 1. *Si Miao Wan*	1. *Golden Rose* (ETHP) 2. *Unlocking Formula* + *Drain Dampness* (HC)
Blood stagnation	Fixed, sharp pain in the lumbar region, aggravated at night and by pressure, difficulty in turning and moving; dark purple tongue body, uneven pulse	Promote blood circulation to remove blood stasis, regulate qi to stop pain	Classical Formulas: 1. *Huo Luo Xiao Ling Dan* 2. *Shu Jing San* Patent Medicines: 1. *Shu Jin He Luo Pian* 2. *Qi Li San*	1. *Meridian Passage* (Jade and K'an) 2. *TR-797* (Pro) 3. *New Resinall K* (HC)

Type	Manifestations	Treatment Principle	Chinese Formula	U.S. Formula and Manufacturer
Kidney qi deficiency	Lingering dull pain with soreness and weakness, aggravated after action, alleviated by rest, preference for pressure and kneading, weakness of the knees; kidney yin deficiency, restlessness, insomnia, dry mouth and throat, flushed cheeks, feverish sensation in the palms and soles; red tongue body, scanty coating, wiry thin and rapid pulse; kidney yang deficiency,: pale complexion, cold limbs, lassitude shortness of breath; pale tongue body, deep and thready pulse	Warm and tonify kidney yang, nourish and tonify kidney yin	Classical Formulas: Kidney yin deficiency 1. *Zuo Gui Wan* Kidney yang deficiency 1. *Jin Gui Shen Qi Wan* 2. *You Gui Wan* Patent Medicines: Kidney yin deficiency 1. *Zuo Gui Wan* Kidney yang deficiency 1. *Jin Gui Shen Qi Wan* 2. *You Gui Wan*	Kidney yin deficiency 1. *Quiet Contemplative* (Jade) 2. *Nine Flavor Tea* (HC) Kidney yang deficiency 1. *LI-487* (Pro) 2. *BO-163* (Pro) 3. *Dynamic Warrior* (Jade and K'an) 4. *MA-511* (Pro)

Menopausal Syndrome

Menopause refers to the inability of the female ovaries to ovulate and produce estrogen. Menopause usually occurs in women in their late forties to early fifties. The onset of menopause is marked by irregular menstruation, which is then followed by cessation of menstruation. It is often accompanied by symptoms that include hot flashes, abnormal perspiration, restlessness, irritability, heart palpitations, insomnia, dizziness, tinnitus, lumbar soreness, weakness of the knees, edema, loose stool, and unusual emotions.

Etiology and pathology

1. Kidney yin deficiency
2. Kidney yang deficiency

Differentiation and treatment

U.S. formulas that can be used in all types include *ME-523* (Pro) and *Two Immortals* (HC).

Type	Manifestations	Treatment Principle	Chinese Formula	U.S. Formula and Manufacturer
Kidney yin deficiency	Dizziness, tinnitus, paroxysmal fever in the face, perspiration, dysphoria with feverish sensations in the palms and soles of the feet, soreness of the lower back and knees, early menstrual cycle or irregular menstrual cycle, profuse or scanty bright red menstrual flow, dry and itchy skin, dry mouth, constipation, scanty yellow urine; red tongue body with scanty coating, thin and rapid pulse	Tonify yin, suppress yang, and regulate Chong and Ren channels	Classical Formulas: 1. *Zuo Gui Yin* + *Zhi shou wu, Gui ban* Patent Medicines: 1. *Qi Ju Di Huang Wan* 2. *Tian Wang Bu Xin Dan* 3. *Liu Wei Di Huang Wan*	1. *Ease Journey-Yin* (WT) 2. *Female Treasure* (WT) 3. *Nine Flavor Tea* (HC) 4. *Energy L* (ETHP) *Note:* For disharmony between heart and kidney, add *Celestial Emperor's Blend* (K'an) or *Heavenly Empress* (WT). For presence of liver qi stagnation, add *Relaxed Wanderer* (Jade and K'an) or other *Xiao Yao Wan* equivalent.
Kidney yang deficiency	Dark complexion, fatigue, intolerance of cold, cold extremities, soreness and coldness of the lower back and knees, poor appetite, abdominal distention, loose stool, heavy, pale menstrual flow or metrorrhagia and metrostaxis, general edema, frequent nocturia or urinary incontinence, clear thin leukorrhea; pale tongue body, thin, white coating, deep, thready and weak pulse	Warm and tonify kidney yang	Classical Formulas: 1. *You Gui Wan* + *Li Zhong Wan*	1. *Ease Journey-Yang* (WT) + *Purge Cold* (TTT) 2. *Energy D* (ETHP) 3. *Astra Essence* (HC) *Note:* For damp cold, add *Dynamic Warrior* (Jade and K'an) and *Water Way* (K'an).

Morning Sickness

Morning sickness is a common complaint among pregnant women, usually experienced during the first trimester. Symptoms include nausea, vomiting, loss of appetite, and dizziness. Severe cases can emaciate the pregnant woman and lead to other disorders.

Etiology and pathology

1. Spleen and stomach qi deficiency
2. Hyperfunction of the Chong meridian
3. Liver blood deficiency
4. Liver yang hyperactivity

Differentiation and treatment

Clinically, there are two types of morning sickness. Treatment focuses on directing rebellious qi downward, harmonizing and tonifying the middle jiao, and stopping vomiting. U.S. formulas that can be used in all types include *Stomach Tabs* (HC), *Soothe the Center* (TTT), *Ease Digestion Formula* (GFCH), and *Ping Wei San Plus* (ETHP).

Type	Manifestations	Treatment Principle	Chinese Formula	U.S. Formula and Manufacturer
Spleen and stomach deficiency	Nausea and vomiting of liquid or undigested food immediately after eating, poor appetite, lassitude, somnolence; pale tongue body with white coating, slippery, slow pulse	Tonify spleen and stomach, direct the rebellious qi downward	Classical Formulas: 1. *Xiang Sha Liu Jun Zi Tang* 2. *Xiao Yao San* 3. *Ping Wei San* Patent Medicines: 1. *Xiang Sha Liu Jun Zi Wan* 2. *Xiao Yao Wan*	1. *Six Gentlemen* (HC) 2. *Ping Wei San Plus* (ETHP) 3. *Six Gentlemen Formula* (GFCH) 4. *GI-335* (Pro)
Disharmony between liver and stomach	Vomiting of bitter or sour liquid, epigastric fullness and distention with hypochondriac pain, frequent belching and sighing, dizziness; slightly yellow tongue coating, slippery, wiry pulse	Harmonize the liver and stomach	Classical Formulas: 1. *Chai Hu Shu Gan San* 2. *Dan Zhi Xiao Yao San* Patent Medicines: 1. *Shu Gan Wan* 2. *Li Gan* 3. *Li Dan*	1. *Shu Gan* (HC) 2. *Women's Relaxing* (ETHP) 3. *Break Into a Smile* (TTT) 4. *Ping Wei San Plus* (ETHP) 5. *PM-637* (Pro) 6. *Harmonize Liver-Spleen* (CMS)

Mumps

Mumps is an acute infectious disease that attacks the parotid glands. It is clinically characterized by fever, pain, and swelling in the parotid region. It occurs throughout the year but most frequently in the winter and spring. Mumps can affect individuals of all ages, but usually children from five to fifteen years of age. While the prognosis of this disease is usually good, it may be complicated, in some cases, by orchitis or meningoencephalitis.

Etiology and pathology

In TCM, mumps is caused by the invasion of epidemic wind heat pathogens.

1. Wind heat pathogen either blocks the Shaoyang meridians or invades the Jueyin meridians.
2. Toxic heat enters into ying and blood and attacks the heart and liver.

Differentiation and treatment

U.S. formulas that can be used in all types include *Clear Heat* (HC) and *Mountain Sophora* (ETHP).

Type	Manifestations	Treatment Principle	Chinese Formula	U.S. Formula and Manufacturer
Wind heat	Slight chills and fever, enlargement of one or both parotids, difficulty in chewing, red throat; red tongue body, thin white coating, or thin slightly yellow coating	Disperse wind heat, relieve the exterior, detoxify	Classical Formulas: 1. *Yin Qiao San* Patent Medicines 1. *Yin Chiao Jie Du Wan* 2. *Sang Ju Pian* 3. *Ling Qiao Jie Du Pian*	1. *Prime Response* (Jade) 2. *Yin Chiao Formula* (GFCH) 3. *Initial Defense* (K'an) 4. *Expel Wind-Heat* (TTT) 5. *CO-197* (Pro) 6. *Phlogisticlean* (CMS)
Toxic heat	High fever, restlessness, headache, thirst, poor appetite or vomiting, feverish sensation, pain and swelling in the parotid region aggravated by pressure, difficulty opening the mouth, chewing, and swallowing food, sore throat, constipation; red tongue body, yellow coating, slippery and rapid pulse	Clear heat and toxins, resolve the swelling	Classical Formulas: 1. *Pu Ji Xiao Du Yin* Patent Medicines: 1. *Niu Huang Jie Du Pian* 2. *Niu Huang Shang Qing Wan*	1. *Purge Heat* (CMS) 2. *Viola Clear Fire Formula* (GFCH) 3. *Five Detox* (LLHP) 4. *CoptiDetox* (K'an)

Obesity

Obesity refers to body weight 15 percent above normal for a given height. (Overweight is 10 percent above normal; gross obesity is 20 percent or more above normal weight.) Chinese medicine has a lengthy tradition in both treating and preventing obesity.

Etiology and pathology

1. Middle jiao hyperactivity
2. Damp phlegm accumulation in middle jiao
3. Stress, leading to irregular eating and/or lack of exercise
4. Constitution

Differentiation and treatment

In TCM there are four types of obesity. Treatment is directed toward transforming damp and phlegm by moving and invigorating qi flow and clearing stomach heat. U.S. formulas that can be used in all types include *Astra Diet Tea* (HC), *Poria 15 Formula* (GFCH), and *Cleansing Formula* (ETHP).

Type	Manifestations	Treatment Principle	Chinese Formula	U.S. Formula and Manufacturer
Middle jiao hyperactivity	Overweight, excessive hunger, overeating, cravings for greasy and spicy food, red face, loud voice; red tongue body with yellow coating, slippery, rapid pulse	Clear stomach heat and eliminate fire	Classical Formulas: 1. *Qing Wei San* Patent Medicines: 1. *Huang Lian Shang Qing Pian*	1. *Gentle Senna* (HC) 2. *Copticlear* (K'an) 3. *Morning Glory* (ETHP)
Damp phlegm accumulation	Overweight, puffy looking, lethargy, fatigue, poor appetite, bland taste, menstrual disorders in females, impotence in males; flabby tongue body with toothmarks, deep, slow, slippery pulse	Disperse damp and transform phlegm	Classical Formulas: 1. *Er Chen Tang* 2. *Liu Jun Zi Tang* 3. *Ling Gui Zhu Gan Tang* Patent Medicines: 1. *Bojianmi Tea* 2. *Er Chen Wan* 3. *Xiang Sha Liu Jun Zi Wan*	1. *Astra 18 Diet* (HC) 2. *Prosperous Farmer* (Jade and K'an) 3. *Purge Phlegm* (CMS) 4. *Green Xiao Yao San* (ETHP)

Type	Manifestations	Treatment Principle	Chinese Formula	U.S. Formula and Manufacturer
Blood stasis in meridians	Overweight, chest and flank pain, palpitations, dizziness; dark red to purple tongue body with thin white coating, deep or choppy pulse	Invigorate the blood flow and dredge the meridians	Classical Formulas: 1. *Gui Zhi Fu Ling Wan* 2. *Dan Shen Yin* 3. *Tong Yu Jian* Patent Medicines: 1. *Yun Nan Bai Yao* 2. *Tong Jing Wan*	1. *Crampbark Plus* (HC) 2. *Women's Palace* (Jade) 3. *Red Stirring* (TTT) 4. *Utrus-A* (LLHP)
Constitutional	Overweight with family history of obesity, various types of water retention, either damp heat or cold damp	Promote water metabolism	Classical Formulas: 1. *Wu Pi Yin* (cold damp) 2. *San Ren Tang* (damp heat) Patent Medicines: 1. *Bojianmi Tea* 2. *Green Tea*	1. *DI-221* (Pro) 2. *Drain Dampness* (HC)

Premenstrual Syndrome

Premenstrual syndrome (PMS) is a group of symptoms that manifests one to fourteen days prior to menstruation, usually one week before, and typically ceases one to two days into the menstrual period. Its etiology remains unclear in Western medicine, though estrogen-progesterone imbalance, vitamin deficiencies, hypoglycemia, prostaglandins, and psychological factors are considered possible causes. The most common symptoms include breast swelling and tenderness, food cravings and compulsive eating, bloating and water retention, headaches, and moodiness. More severe symptoms include vomiting, boils on the skin, vertigo and fainting, and paresthesias (tingling) of the hands and feet. PMS is thought to occur in up to 50 percent of menstruating women, with 95 percent of them aged eighteen to forty years. In TCM, it is known as *Yue Jing Bing*, meaning "menstrual disorder."

Etiology and pathology

The liver and kidney are the main organs involved in PMS.

1. Liver qi stagnation leads to *shu xie* dysfunction, resulting an overcontrolled spleen and stomach, which in turn results in damp accumulation
2. Liver and kidney yin deficiency in which there is a failure of nourishment

Differentiation and treatment

PMS can manifest as excess, deficient, or a combination of the two. How it manifests depends on the individual's constitution. Treatment is directed at the causal factor, the root, as well as the manifestations, or branches. U.S. formulas that can be used in all types include *PM-637* (Pro).

Type	Manifestations	Treatment Principle	Chinese Formula	U.S. Formula and Manufacturer
Liver qi stagnation	Distending pain in the breasts and costal-hypochondriac region prior to menses, colic or distending pain in the lower abdomen after menstruation starts, scanty red flow with dark red, purple, or brown clots, headache, irritability; red-tipped tongue body with thin yellow coating, thready, choppy, or wiry pulse	Regulate liver qi, activate blood circulation	Classical Formulas: 1. *Xiao Yao San* 2. *Chai Hu Shu Gan San* 3. *Dang Gui Shao Yao San* Patent Medicines: 1. *Xiao Yao Wan* 2. *Shu Gan Wan* 3. *Fu Fang Dang Gui Pian* 4. *Dang Gui Shu*	1. *Relaxed Wanderer* (Jade and K'an) 2. *Woman's Balance* (HC) 3. *Smooth Passage* (TTT) (with more GI symptoms) 4. *Free Flow* (WT) (if much pain present) 5. *Disperse Qi* (CMS) 6. *Shu Xie Tea* (ETHP) 7. *Smooth Cycle* (CHC) 8. *Liver-Qi Pacifier* (LLHP) (if much pain present) 9. *Xiao Yao Wan Plus* (GFCH) (if heat present) 10. *Bupleurum and Tang Kuei Formula* (GFCH)

Type	Manifestations	Treatment Principle	Chinese Formula	U.S. Formula and Manufacturer
Liver and kidney yin deficiency	Dull pain or discomfort in costal-hypochondriac region prior to and during menstruation, distending, spasmodic pain in lower abdomen after menstruation, scanty dark-red or pale menstrual flow, dizziness, tinnitus, flushed face, afternoon feverish sensations, dry mouth, dry skin, brittle nails; red tongue body with little coating, thin or wiry pulse	Nourish liver and kidney yin	Classical Formulas: 1. *Liu Wei Di Huang Wan* 2. *Zhi Bai Di Huang Wan* 3. *Yi Guan Jian* Patent Medicines: 1. *Liu Wei Di Huang Wan* 2. *Zhi Bai Di Huang Wan* 3. *Ba Zhen Yi Mu Wan* 4. *Zuo Gui Wan*	1. *Fertile Garden + Nine Flavor Tea* (HC) 2. *Tonify Moisture* (CMS) 3. *Nourish the Root* (TTT) 4. *Nourish Essence Formula* (GFCH) 5. *Quiet Contemplative* (Jade and K'an) 6. *Energy L* (ETHP)

Rhinitis and Sinusitis

Rhinitis involves the inflammation of the nasomembrane and is characterized by excessive nasal discharge, congestion, and edema. Sinusitis involves inflammation of the nasal sinuses and manifests as sinus pain and pressure, congestion, and increased nasal discharge. In TCM, both fall under the category of *Biyan*, which means "thick and sticky nasal discharge," and includes loss of the sense of smell. Rhinitis and sinusitis are considered together in TCM.

Etiology and pathology

The lungs are the main organ system involved, as the lungs open into the nose.

1. Wind cold invasion leading to lung qi blockage
2. Wind dry heat invasion leading to lung qi blockage and nasal passage dryness
3. Uprising of liver/gallbladder heat, disturbing the fluid-dispersing function of the lungs

Differentiation and treatment

TCM treats rhinitis and sinusitis by clearing the lungs and nasal cavities. U.S. formulas that can be used in all types include *Bi Yan Pian* (K'an), *Nasal Tabs* (HC), and *NA-551* (Pro).

Type	Manifestations	Treatment Principle	Chinese Formula	U.S. Formula and Manufacturer
Wind cold	Severe nasal obstruction, nasal itching, profuse thin white or clear and colorless nasal discharge, sneezing, headache, chills, fever; normal tongue body with thin white coating, floating pulse	Disperse wind cold, open nasal passages	Classical Formulas: 1. *Cang Er Zi San* 2. *Jing Fang Bai Du San* 3. *Chuan Xiong Cha Tiao San* Patent Medicines: 1. *Pe Min Kan Wan*	1. *Xanthium Relieve Surface* (HC) 2. *AL-113* (Pro) 3. *Purge External Wind* (CMS) 4. *Jade Screen and Xanthium Formula* (GFCH) 5. *X. Plus* (ETHP) 6. *Allergease* (LLHP)
Wind dry heat	Nasal dryness, nasal congestion with scanty yellow discharge and/or bloody discharge, fever and chills, cough, sore, dry throat; red tongue tip with thin yellow coating, floating, rapid pulse	Disperse and clear wind dry heat; restore the lung's xanjiang function	Classical Formulas: 1. *Yin Qiao San* 2. *Ju Hua Cha Tiao San* 3. *Sang Ju Yin* 4. *Sang Xing Tang* Patent Medicines: 1. *Yin Chiao Jie Du Pian* 2. *Sang Yu Pian* 3. *Bi Yan Pian* 4. *Bi Yan Wan*	1. *Astra C + Yin Chiao Jin* (HC) 2. *CO-197 + HA-341* (Pro) 3. *Yin Chiao Formula* (GFCH) + *Light Clearing* (ETHP) 4. *Prime Response* (Jade) 5. *B. Plus + Isatis Compound* (ETHP) 6. *Purge Heat* (CMS)
Liver/ gallbladder heat	Purulent nasal discharge with headache, red and painful eyes, hypochondriac pain, anger, irritability, bitter taste in the mouth, nausea, jaundiced complexion; red tongue sides with yellow greasy coating, rapid, wiry pulse	Clear liver/ gallbladder heat	Classical Formulas: 1. *Long Dan Xie Gan Tang* 2. *Hao Qin Qing Dan Tang* 3. *Ling Yang Jiao Tang* Patent Medicines: 1. *Long Dan Xie Gan Wan* 2. *Bi Yan Pian*	1. *Coptis Purge Fire* (HC) 2. *Quell Fire* (Jade and K'an) 3. *Purge Internal Wind* (CMS) 4. *Q.B.Y.* (ETHP) 5. *Gentiana Drain Fire Formula* (GFCH)

Smoking Addiction

The knowledge that smoking is hazardous to their health prods many smokers to seek help in ridding themselves of their addiction. Together with acupuncture, Chinese herbal medicine can help smokers quit. Chinese herbal treatment is directed toward decreasing the craving for nicotine, strengthening will power, detoxification, and changing the taste in the mouth, which leads to a cessation of smoking.

Etiology and pathology

1. Heart and lung qi deficiency
2. Lung and kidney yin deficiency
3. Yin deficiency with yang rising
4. Spleen and stomach deficiency
5. Stomach damp heat

Differentiation and treatment

U.S. formulas that can be used in all types are *Clear Air* (HC), *White Flower* (ETHP), and *Stop Smoking Tea* (China).

Type	Manifestations	Treatment Principle	Chinese Formula	U.S. Formula and Manufacturer
Heart and lung qi deficiency	Long-term heavy smoker, cold and weak constitution, weak upper jiao that feels stronger with smoking, cough, wheezing, chest congestion, palpitations, shortness of breath, anxiety, dream-disturbed sleep; pale and flabby tongue, weak and scattered pulse; symptoms improve with smoking	Tonify heart and lung qi	Classical Formulas: 1. *Bao Yuan Tang* Patent Medicines: 1. *Li Fei* 2. *Stop Smoking Tea*	1. *Ginseng and Gecko Herbal Formula* (HC) 2. *Energy A* (ETHP) 3. *Open the Heart* (TTT) 4. *Ginseng and Astragalus Formula* (GFCH)

Type	Manifestations	Treatment Principle	Chinese Formula	U.S. Formula and Manufacturer
Liver and kidney yin deficiency with empty heat	Long-term light smoker, heat and weak constitution, strong cravings, dull headaches, dizziness, tinnitus, insomnia or dream-disturbed sleep, flushed cheeks, blurred vision, night sweats, nocturnal emmissions, light menses or amenorrhea; red tongue body with little coating, rapid, thready pulse; symptoms worse with smoking	Nourish liver and kidney yin, clear deficient heat	Classical Formulas: 1. *Da Bu Yin Wan* 2. *Liu Wei Di Huang Wan* 3. *Zuo Gui Wan* Patent Medicines: 1. *Liu Wei Di Huang Wan* 2. *Zhi Bai Di Huang Wan* 3. *Zuo Gui Wan*	1. *Nine Flavor Tea* (HC) 2. *Energy L* (ETHP) 3. *Nourish the Root* (TTT) 4. *Quiet Contemplative* (Jade and K'an) 5. *Nourish Essence Formula* (GFCH)
Spleen and stomach deficiency	Weak gastrointestinal system, cravings increased when hungry, discomfort in epigastrium, poor appetite, loose stools, abdominal distention, fatigue, heavy head sensation; pale, flabby tongue body, empty pulse; symptoms improve with smoking	Tonify spleen and stomach	Classical Formulas: 1. *Bu Zhong Yi Qi Tang* 2. *Shen Ling Bai Zhu San* 3. *Liu Jun Zi Tang* Patent Medicines: 1. *Bu Zhong Yi Qi Wan* 2. *Shen Ling Bai Zhu Wan* 3. *Liu Jun Zi Wan*	1. *Six Gentlemen* (HC) 2. *Source Qi* (HC) 3. *Energy K* (ETHP) 4. *Soothe the Center* (TTT) 5. *Prosperous Farmer* (Jade and K'an) 6. *Astragalus Formula* (GFCH)
Stomach damp heat	Damp heat constitution, heavy smoker, craving increases after meals, heartburn, belching, stomachache worse with heat, thirst for cold drinks; red tongue body with thick, yellow, sticky coating, tense, rapid pulse	Clear damp heat	Classical Formulas: 1. *Qing Wei San* Patent Medicines: 1. *Huang Lian Shang Qing Pian* 2. *Niu Huang Jie Du Pian* 3. Green tea	1. *Gentle Senna* (HC) 2. *Copticlear* (K'an)

Sore Throat

Sore throat usually appears as a secondary condition that manifests as a symptom of a common cold, flu, or problems associated with eating excessive amounts of spicy foods or consuming too much coffee or alcohol. In these cases, it generally appears with fever, chills, headache, cough, sputum, or epigastric distress. Sore throat is also indicated in tonsillitis, pharyngitis, and laryngitis. Sore throat can also manifest by itself as a primary condition. In TCM, sore throat is called *Hou E* and *Hou Bi*.

Etiology and pathology

The lung, stomach, and kidney are the primary organs involved.

1. Wind heat invades the lung and moves through the trachea to the throat
2. Accumulated stomach heat in which heat travels through the esophagus to the throat
3. Kidney yin deficiency in which there is a failure of the upward moistening function which leads to deficient fire flaring up from the kidney to the kidney meridian to the throat

Differentiation and treatment

Clinically, sore throat is differentiated into three types. Treatment is directed toward dispersing heat, nourishing yin, and inducing deficient fire down to the root. U.S. formulas that can be used in all types include *Clear Lung* (CHC), *Strengthen Lung* (CMS), *Pinellia Phlegm Dispersing Formula* (K'an), and *Jade Screen* (ETHP).

Type	Manifestations	Treatment Principle	Chinese Formula	U.S. Formula and Manufacturer
Wind heat	Abrupt onset of congested and sore throat with fever and chills, headache, cough, hoarse voice; red tongue tip with thin yellow or white coating, floating, rapid pulse	Release the exterior, clear heat	Classical Formulas: 1. *Shu Feng Qing Re Tang* 2. *Yin Qiao San* 3. *Sang Ju Yin* Patent Medicines: 1. *Lu Shen Wan* 2. *Yin Chiao Jie Du Pian* 3. *Sang Ju Pian* 4. *Chuan Xin Lian Kang Yan Pian*	1. *Yin Chao Jin* + *Clear Heat* (HC) 2. *Light Clearing* (ETHP) 3. *Prime Response* (Jade) 4. *Initial Defense* (K'an) 5. *Expel Wind Heat* (TTT) 6. *CO-197* (Pro) 7. *Yin Chiao Formula* (GFCH)

Type	Manifestations	Treatment Principle	Chinese Formula	U.S. Formula and Manufacturer
Accumulated stomach and lung heat	Red, swollen, and sore throat with fever, thirst for cold drinks, halitosis, cough with sticky, yellow sputum, difficulty swallowing, constipation, concentrated urine; red tongue with yellow coating, rapid, forceful pulse	Clear toxic heat, relieve soreness and swelling of the throat	Classical Formulas: 1. *Qing Yan Li Ge Tang* 2. *Wu Wei Xiao Du Yin* Patent Medicines: 1. *Qing Qi Hua Tan Wan* 2. *Lu Shen Wan*	1. *Isatis Gold + Coptis Purge Fire Formula* (HC) 2. *Mountain Sophora* (ETHP) 3. *Five Detox* (LLHP) 4. *Detox Compound* (CHC) 5. *Phlogisticlean* (CMS) 6. *Viola Clear Fire Formula* (GFCH)
Kidney yin deficiency with heat	Gradual onset of slightly red and mild sore throat, soreness worse at night, soreness that comes and goes, sore when swallowing, low-grade fever or afternoon fever, heat sensation in palms and soles; thin red tongue body with little coating, thready and rapid pulse	Nourish kidney yin	Classical Formulas: 1. *Zhi Bai Di Huang Wan* 2. *Liu Wei Di Huang Wan* Patent Medicines: 1. *Zhi Bai Di Huang Wan* 2. *Liu Wei Di Huang Wan* 3. *Qing Yin Wan*	1. *Nine Flavor Tea* (HC) 2. *Energy L + Pang Da Hai Com-pound* (ETHP) 3. *Nourish the Root* (TTT) 4. *Quiet Contemplative* (Jade and K'an) 5. *Nourish Essence Formula* (GFCH) 6. *Tonify Moisture* (CMS) 7. *Full Circle* (CHC)

Tinnitus and Deafness

Tinnitus and deafness are both auditory disorders. Tinnitus is characterized by the subjective experience of noise in the ears, such as ringing, rumbling, or buzzing, while deafness is loss of hearing, either partial or complete. Tinnitus can be a precursor of deafness. Because in TCM these two disorders share a similar etiology, pathogenesis, and treatment, they are discussed together.

Etiology and pathology

Tinnitus and deafness can have either of two general etiologies: deficiency or excess. The kidney and the liver/gallbladder organ pair are the principal organs involved in tinnitus and deafness.

1. Deficiency
   - Kidney qi or essence deficiency that results in an inability to nourish the ear
   - Kidney yin deficiency in which empty yang rises to disturb the ear and interfere with its functioning
2. Excess
   - Rage, anger, stress, or fright that stirs liver/gallbladder fire and leads to upward disturbance that blocks the meridians of the ear
   - Damp heat, phlegm, or liver yang excess that leads to upward disturbance that blocks the meridians around the ear

Differentiation and treatment

Treatment is directed toward nourishing the yin essence in the case of deficiency and restraining the yang in the case of excess. U.S. formulas that can be used in all types include *G. Plus* (ETHP).

Type	Manifestations	Treatment Principle	Chinese Formula	U.S. Formula and Manufacturer
Deficient type	Protracted deafness, intermittent low-pitched, buzzing tinnitus, exacerbated by strain, relieved by pressure and rest, possible dizziness, low backache, weak lower limbs, nocturnal emission, excessive leukorrhea; pale, thin, or flabby tongue body, thready weak pulse	Nourish yin essence or tonify qi and yang	Classical Formulas: Yin deficiency 1. *Er Long Zuo Ci Wan* 2. *Liu Wei Di Huang Wan* Yang deficiency 1. *Bu Gu Zhi Wan* 2. *Jin Gui Shen Qi Wan* Patent Medicines: 1. *Er Long Zuo Ci Wan* 2. *Liu Wei Di Huang Wan* 3. *Golden Book Tea*	1. *Astra Essence* (HC) 2. *Quiet Contemplative* (Jade and K'an) 3. *Eight Immortals Formula* (GFCH) 4. *Energy L* (ETHP) (yin essence deficiency) 5. *Nourish the Root* (TTT) (yin essence deficiency) 6. *Strengthen the Root* (TTT) (yang qi deficiency) 7. *Energy D* (ETHP) (yang qi deficiency)

Type	Manifestations	Treatment Principle	Chinese Formula	U.S. Formula and Manufacturer
Excess type	Sudden deafness, distending sensation and constant ringing in the ear of high pitch or loud sound, like thunder, a roar, or a cicada chirp, ringing unrelieved by pressure, possible flushed face, irritability, dry mouth, chest congestion with sputum, dry mouth; red tongue with sticky yellow coating, slippery, rapid pulse	Clear and drain the liver/ gallbladder damp heat	Classical Formulas: 1. *Long Dan Xie Gan Tang* 2. *Qing Qi Hua Tan Wan* Patent Medicines: 1. *Long Dan Xie Gan Wan* 2. *Qing Qi Hua Tan Wan* (*Clean Air Tea*)	1. *Coptis Purge Fire* (HC) 2. *Release Constraint + Drain Fire* (TTT) 3. *Quell Fire* (Jade and K'an) 4. *R.D.Y.* (ETHP) 5. *Detox Compound* (CHC) 6. *LD-477* (Pro) 7. *Gentiana Drain Fire Formula* (GFCH) 8. *Purge Damp Heat* (CMS) 9. *Pinellia Phlegm Dispersing Formula* (K'an)

Urticaria

Urticaria is a skin condition characterized by red or pale slightly raised wheals that are flat-topped and may itch severely. The wheals can resemble measles or be as large as broad beans. Because it can be precipitated by exposure to wind and involves itching skin, urticaria is called "wind wheal" in TCM. And because it comes and goes, it is also known as "hidden rash."

Etiology and pathology

The lung, stomach, and large intestine are the main organs involved.

1. Dampness in the skin and muscles attacked by wind damp or wind heat
2. Damp heat toxin in the stomach and large intestine attacked by wind
3. Parasites or allergies

Differentiation and treatment

Clinically, there are three types of urticaria. Treatment is directed toward dispersing wind and damp, eliminating heat toxins, and activating blood. U.S. formulas that can be used in all types include *Skin Balance* (HC).

Type	Manifestations	Treatment Principle	Chinese Formula	U.S. Formula and Manufacturer
Wind heat	Bright red rash with severe itching, vesicles of various sizes that erupt and ooze, symptoms may be aggravated by changes in weather; floating and rapid pulse	Disperse wind, clear heat	Classical Formulas 1. *Xiao Feng San* 2. *Yin Qiao San* + *Jing Fang Bai Du San* Patent Medicines: 1. *Yin Chiao Jie Du Pian*	1. *Clear Heat* + *Yin Chao San* (HC) 2. *Glorious Sea* + *Expel Wind Heat* (TTT) 3. *Skin-Cleanser* (LLHP) 4. *Clear Lungs* (CHC) 5. *Purge External Wind* (CMS) 6. *Prime Response* + *Prime Rescue* (Jade) 7. *Initial Defense* + *Dispel Invasion* (K'an) 8. *CO-197* (Pro)
Wind damp	White or light-colored rash accompanied by heaviness of the body, precipitated or exacerbated by wet weather, improved with dry weather; white or sticky white tongue coating, floating and slow pulse	Disperse wind and transform damp	Classical Formulas: 1. *Huo Xiang Zheng Qi San* 2. *Huo Po Xia Ling Tang* Patent Medicines: 1. *Huo Xiang Zheng Qi Wan*	1. *Prime Relief* (Jade) 2. *Early Comfort* (K'an) 3. *Drain Fields* (TTT) 4. *R.D.A.* (ETHP)
Damp heat toxin	Bright red rash accompanied by abdominal and epigastric pain, constipation, or diarrhea, may be precipitated by certain foods or overeating; sticky yellow tongue coating, slippery and rapid pulse	Clear toxic heat, drain damp	Classical Formulas: 1. *Fang Feng Tong Sheng San* Patent Medicines: 1. *Fang Feng Tong Sheng Wan* 2. *Huang Lian Shang Qing Wan*	1. *Coptis Purge Fire Formula* + *Skin Balance* (HC) 2. *Flavor 21* (ETHP) 3. *Coptis Relieve Toxicity Formula* (GFCH) 4. *Clear Lustre* (TTT) 5. *Si Miao Wan* + *Five Detox* (LLHP) 6. *Clear Skin* (CHC) 7. *Purge Heat* + *Purge Damp Heat* (CMS) 8. *LD-477* (Pro)

Urinary Tract Infection

Urinary tract infection (UTI) is characterized by burning, frequent, painful, and difficult urination, usually accompanied by lower back pain. In TCM, UTI fits into the category of *Lin*, or "urinary disturbance," syndrome. It is associated with disorder of the urinary bladder in controlling urinary discharge chiefly caused by an attack of pathogenic damp heat and dysfunction of the Zang and Fu organs.

Etiology and pathology

1. Attack of the bladder by damp heat
2. Spleen deficiency which leads to sinking of qi of middle jiao
3. Stagnation of liver qi
4. Kidney deficiency

Differentiation and treatment

U.S. formulas that can be used in all types include *Lower Burner* (Jade) and *Jin Qian Cao Stone Formula* (HC).

Type	Manifestations	Treatment Principle	Chinese Formula	U.S. Formula and Manufacturer
Retention of damp heat in the bladder	Frequent, urgent, burning, and painful urination, scanty, dark urine, hematuria, suprapubic and low back pain, chills and fever, bitter taste in the mouth, dry stool; red tongue body, yellow greasy coating, soft and rapid pulse	Clear damp heat, promote diuresis to stop the stranguria (painful urination)	Classical Formulas: 1. *Ba Zheng San* Patent Medicines: 1. *Jin Qian Cao Chong Ji* 2. *Shi Lin Tong Pian*	1. *UI-821* (Pro) 2. *Akebia Relieving Formula* (K'an) 3. *Jin Qian Cao Stone Formula* (HC) 4. *Akebia Moist Heat Formula* (HC) *Note:* For pathogen in the shaoyang with chills, fever, bitter taste in the mouth, nausea, or vomiting, add *AL-113* (Pro), or *Minor Bupleurum* (K'an).

Type	Manifestations	Treatment Principle	Chinese Formula	U.S. Formula and Manufacturer
Spleen deficiency	Dripping urination, bearing-down sensation in the lower abdomen aggravated with exertion, pale complexion; pale tongue body, thin and weak pulse	Tonify spleen qi	Classical Formulas: 1. *Bu Zhong Yi Qi Wan* 2. *Bu Zhong Yi Qi Tang* Patent Medicines: 1. *Bu Zhong Yi Qi Wan* 2. *Bu Zhong Yi Qi Tang*	1. *Arouse Vigor* (Jade and K'an) 2. *Source Qi* (HC) 3. *EN-261* (Pro)
Liver qi stagnation	Erratic discharge of urine, dribbling urination, distention or pain in the lower abdomen; thin, white tongue coating, deep and wiry pulse	Soothe the liver to relieve the stagnant liver qi	Classical Formulas: 1. *Xiao Yao Wan* 2. *Xiao Yao San* Patent Medicines 1. *Xiao Yao Wan* 2. *Xiao Yao San*	1. *PM-637* (Pro) + *Jin Qian Cao Stone Formula* (HC) 2. *Woman's Balance* (HC) + *Jin Qian Cao Stone Formula* (HC) 3. *Coptis Purge Fire Formula* (HC) + *Jin Qian Cao Stone Formula* (HC) 4. *Quell Fire* (Jade and K'an) + *Jin Qian Cao Stone Formula* (HC) 5. *CY-207* (Pro) + *Jin Qian Cao Stone Formula* (HC)
Kidney deficiency	Lingering, intermittent urinary disturbance, usually occurring after overstrain, soreness, and weakness of the loins and knees, fatigue; kidney yin deficiency/ if flushed cheeks, feverish sensation in the palms, soles of feet and chest; red tongue body, thin and rapid pulse; kidney yang deficiency/ if pale face; pale tongue body, deep, slow, and weak pulse	Strengthen and consolidate kidney qi, tonify kidney yin, reinforce kidney yang	Patent Medicines: Kidney qi deficiency 1. *Wu Bi Shan Yao Wan* Kidney yin deficiency 1. *Zhi Bai Di Huang Wan or Liu Wei Di Huang Wan + Zhi zi, Mu dan pi* Kidney yang deficiency 1. *Jin Gui Shen Qi Wan or You Gui Wan*	Kidney yin deficiency 1. *Temper Fire* (Jade and K'an) or *Quiet Contemplative* (Jade and K'an) Kidney yang deficiency 1. *Dynamic Warrior* (Jade and K'an) or *Rehmannia 8* (HC) Kidney qi deficiency 1. *R.D.K.* (ETHP)

Xiao Ke (Diabetes)

Xiao Ke is a TCM disease that refers to the clinical manifestations of polyphagia, polydipsia, polyuria, and loss of body weight. It includes diabetes mellitus in Western medicine. In TCM, Xiao Ke is roughly classified as upper xiao, middle xiao, and lower xiao. The *Classified Mature Medica* (1602 A.D.), by Wang Kengtang, says, "Polydipsia belongs to Upper Xiao; polyphagia, Middle Xiao; polyuria, Lower Xiao." Although Xiao Ke is divided into three Xiaos, its pathological root is the same, for it is associated with disorders of the lung, stomach (spleen), and kidney, as well as yin deficiency with its heat and dryness.

Etiology and pathology

1. Improper diet causing damp heat and damaging stomach yin
2. Emotional stress leading to liver qi stagnation, resulting in heat
3. Sexual overstrain internally consuming kidney yin and essence, leading to deficient fire.

Differentiation and treatment

U.S. formulas that can be used in all types include *Eight Immortals Formula* (GFCH).

Type	Manifestations	Treatment Principle	Chinese Formula	U.S. Formula and Manufacturer
Upper Xiao—lung heat and consumption of body fluid	Restlessness, polydipsia, dry mouth and tongue, polyuria; red tip and edge of the tongue, thin, yellow coating, full and rapid pulse	Clear heat and moisten the lungs, promote regeneration of body fluid to stop thirst	Classical Formulas: 1. *Xiao Ke Fang* Patent Medicines: 1. *Shen Mai Yin* 2. *Yu Quan Wan*	1. *Tonify Moisture* (CMS) 2. *Herbal Sentinel-Yin* (TTT) 3. *Wise Jade* (K'an) 4. *Wise Judge* (Jade)
Middle Xiao—stomach fire with consumption of yin	Polyphagia with tendency toward hunger, emaciation, dry stool with constipation; red tongue body, yellow coating, slippery and rapid pulse	Clear the stomach and purge fire, tonify yin, and increase body fluid	Classical Formulas: 1. *Yu Nu Jian* + *Huang lian, Zhi zi* Patent Medicines: 1. *Huang Lian Shang Qing Pian*	1. *Jade Spring* (TTT) 2. *Chemo-Support* (TTT) 3. *Tonify Moisure* (CMS) 4. *TCB14 Trichosanthes Combination* (MG) *Note:* For fire in the stomach and intestines with constipation, add *Smooth Response* (K'an).

Type	Manifestations	Treatment Principle	Chinese Formula	U.S. Formula and Manufacturer
Lower Xiao—kidney yin deficiency	Polyuria with turbid dis-charge, urine sweet in taste, soreness and debility of the lumbar area, dry mouth and lips, feverish sensation of the palms, soles, and chest; red tongue body with scanty coating, deep, thin and rapid pulse	Nourish yin and consolidate the kidney	Classical Formulas: 1. *Liu Wei Di Huang Wan* Patent Medicines: 1. *Liu Wei Di Huang Wan* 2. *Zhi Bai Di Huang Wan*	1. *Quiet Contemplative* (Jade) 2. *Nine Flavor Tea* (HC) 3. *TCB 7 (Cornus Combination)* (MG) 4. *Temper Fire* (Jade and K'an) *Note:* For profuse urination with cloudy urine, add *Restore Integrity* (K'an) or *Firm Vessel* (Jade).
Lower Xiao—deficiency of both yin and yang	Frequent urination with turbid discharge, dark complexion, dry, withered auricle, soreness and weakness of the loins and knees, intolerance of cold, cold limbs; pale tongue body, white coating, deep, thready, and weak pulse	Warm yang, nourish yin, and consolidate the kidney	Classical Formulas: 1. *Jin Gui Shen Qi Wan* Patent Medicines: 1. *Jin Gui Shen Qi Wan* 2. *Suo Quan Wan*	1. *Dynamic Warrior* (Jade and K'an) 2. *Rehmannia 8* (HC) *Note:* The above can be combined with *Restore Integrity* (K'an) or *Firm Vessel* (Jade).

Yin Ting (Uterine Prolapse)

Yin Ting (uterine prolapse) occurs when the uterus slips out of place or the vaginal wall protrudes out of the vagina. In Western terms, the disease corresponds to metroptosis.

Etiology and pathology

The spleen and kidney are the main organs involved in yin ting.

1. Qi deficiency
2. Kidney deficiency
3. Damp heat in the lower jiao

Differentiation and treatment

U.S. formulas that can be used in all types include *Tonify Qi* and *Ease the Muscles* (TTT) and *Tonify Qi* (CMS).

Type	Manifestations	Treatment Principle	Chinese Formula	U.S. Formula and Manufacturer
Qi deficiency	Uterus descending into the vagina or out of the vaginal orifice, aggravated by overstrain, sinking sensation in the lower abdomen, general lassitude, shortness of breath, pale complexion, copious thin white leukorrhea; pale tongue body, thin white coating, weak pulse	Tonify qi, lift yang, and consolidate the uterus	Classical Formulas: 1. *Bu Zhong Yi Qi Tang* Patent Medicines: 1. *Bu Zhong Yi Qi Wan*	1. *Arouse Vigor* (K'an and Jade) 2. *Ginseng and Astragalus Formula* (GFCH) 3. *Energy K* (ETHP) 4. *Consolidate Qi* (CMS) 5. *Astra 8* (HC)
Kidney deficiency	Prolapse of uterus with sinking sensation in the lower abdomen, dizziness, tinnitus, soreness in the lower back and knees, frequent urination, especially at night; slight red tongue body, deep, weak pulse	Tonify kidney qi and consolidate the uterus	Classical Formulas: 1. *Da Bu Yuan Jian + Jin yin zi, Qian shi, Lu jiao jiao, Zi he che*	1. *Unicorn Pearl* (WT) 2. *Astra Essence* (HC) *Note:* Use either of the above together with *Arouse Vigor* (K'an and Jade) or *Ginseng and Astragalus Formula* (GFCH)
Damp heat	Uterine prolapse, uterus protrudes through vaginal orifice, red, swollen, and ulcerated surface with continuous dripping of yellowish fluid, foul-smelling copious yellowish leukorrhea mixed with pus and blood, fever, thirst, dark urine, local burning pain; red tongue body, yellow greasy coating, rapid pulse	Clear damp heat	Classical Formulas: 1. *Long Dan Xie Gan Tang* Patent Medicines: 1. *Long Dan Xie Gan Wan*	1. *Quell Fire* (K'an and Jade) 2. *Gentiana Drain Fire Formula* (GFCH) 3. *Coptis Purge Fire* (HC) 4. *Gentiana Compound* (ETHP)

Yin Yang (Vaginal Itching)

Yin Yang is a TCM disease category that corresponds to pruritus, or intense itching, of the genitalia, including pruritus vulvae and vaginal pruritus. The condition may be accompanied by increased vaginal discharge. In severe cases, the pruritus and pain are unbearable. The disease also corresponds to vulvitis, vaginitis, senile vaginitis, and pruritus vulvae in Western medicine.

Etiology and pathology

1. Downward flow of damp heat
2. Liver and kidney yin deficiency
3. Stagnated fire of the heart and liver

Differentiation and treatment

U.S. formulas that can be used in all types include *Peaceful Sunset* (TTT) and *Purge Damp Heat* (CMS).

Type	Manifestations	Treatment Principle	Chinese Formula	U.S. Formula and Manufacturer
Damp heat	Pruritus vulvae, accompanied by pain in severe cases, profuse yellow and purulent or milky and frothy vaginal discharge with a fetid smell, restlessness, poor sleep, bitter taste in the mouth, fullness in the chest, poor appetite; sticky yellow tongue coating, wiry, rapid pulse	Clear damp heat and stop itching	Classical Formulas: 1. *Bei Xie Shen Shi Tang + Cang zhu, Ku shen, Bai xian pi* 2. *Long Dan Xie Gan Tang* Patent Medicines: 1. *Long Dan Xie Gan Wan*	1. *Drain the Jade Valley* (WT) 2. *Quell Fire* (K'an and Jade) 3. *Gentiana Drain Fire Formula* (GFCH)

Type	Manifestations	Treatment Principle	Chinese Formula	U.S. Formula and Manufacturer
Liver and kidney yin xu	Dryness, burning sensation, and pruritus of the genitalia, scanty, yellow or blood-tinged vaginal discharge, restlessness, heat sensation in the palms, soles, and chest, dizziness, blurred vision, feverish sensation in the face, perspiration, dry mouth with no desire to drink, tinnitus, lumbar soreness; red tongue body with scanty coating, rapid, weak pulse	Tonify yin and relieve itching	Classical Formulas: 1. *Zhi Bai Di Huang Wan + Bai xian pi, Zhi shou wu* 2. *Qi Ju Di Huang Wan + Bai xian pi* Patent Medicines: 1. *Zhi Bai Di Huang Wan*	1. Temper Fire (K'an and Jade) 2. *Rehmannia and Scrophularia* (GFCH) 3. *Q.B.Y.* (ETHP)
Heart and liver stagnated fire	Pruritus of the genitalia, worse at night, distention of the chest, irritability, hot temper, anxiety, poor sleep; red tongue body, yellow coating, wiry and rapid pulse	Soothe the liver and clear the liver fire	Classical Formulas: 1. *Dan Zhi Xiao Yao San + Long chi*	1. *Free Flow* (WT) 2. *Free and Easy Wanderer Plus* (GFCH) 3. *Woman's Balance* (HC)

Yu Syndrome (Depression)

Yu syndrome is, in TCM, a general term for disorders resulting from irregular emotions and stagnation of qi, mostly manifested by emotional depression, distending pain in the hypochondriac regions, hot temper, grief, the subjective sensation of a foreign body stuck in the throat, and insomnia. This condition can be viewed as hysteria, neurosis, depression, anxiety, and panic attacks in Western medicine. Yu syndrome results from emotional injuries which result in depressed liver qi, leading gradually to disharmony of qi activity in the five Zang organs. It can manifest as an excess type, referred to as depressed anger, or a deficient type, called mental depression.

Etiology and pathology

Depressed anger

1. Stagnation of liver qi due to mental stress and emotional stimulation
2. Liver fire caused by long-term liver qi stagnation or liver yin deficiency
3. Stagnation of phlegm misting the pericardium and heart shen

Mental depression

1. Impairment of the mind caused by heart and kidney disconnetion
2. Spleen and heart deficiency, causing qi deficiency and heart shen wandering
3. Kidney yin deficiency leading to a failure to nourish the heart

Differentiation and treatment

U.S. formulas that can be used in all types include *Relaxed Wanderer* (Jade and K'an).

Type	Manifestations	Treatment Principle	Chinese Formula	U.S. Formula and Manufacturer
Liver qi stagnation	Mental depression, deep breathing, frequent sighing, distending pain in the chest and hypochondrium, fullness in the epigastric area, belching, abdominal distention, anorexia, vomiting, abnormal bowel movement, amenorrhea; thin, greasy tongue coating, wiry pulse	Soothe the liver, promote qi circulation to relieve stagnation	Classical Formulas: 1. *Xiao Yao San* Patent Medicines: 1. *Xiao Yao Wan*	1. *Free and Easy Wanderer* (K'an) 2. *Break Into a Smile* (TTT)
Liver fire	Irritability, hot temper, distress of the chest, hypochondriac distention, acid regurgitation, dryness and bitter taste in the mouth, constipation, headache, red eyes, and tinnitus; red tongue body, yellow coating, wiry and rapid pulse	Clear liver fire, soothe liver qi, and regulate the stomach	Classical Formulas: 1. *Dan Zhi Xiao Yao San* + *Zuo Jin Wan*	1. *Woman's Balance* (HC) + *GI 337* (Pro) *Note:* Add *Smooth Response* (K'an) if dry stool present.

Type	Manifestations	Treatment Principle	Chinese Formula	U.S. Formula and Manufacturer
Stagnation of phlegm	Feeling of a foreign body stuck in the throat that is difficult to spit out or swallow down (also known as globus hystericus), oppressive sensation in the chest, hypochondriac pain; greasy white tongue coating, wiry, slippery pulse	Resolve phlegm, promote qi circulation to relieve stagnation	Classical Formulas: 1. *Wen Dan Tang* 2. *Di Tan Tang*	1. *Purge Phlegm* (CMS) 2. *Clear the Soul* + *Break Into a Smile* (TTT)
Impairment of mind	Catatonia, grief and anger without reasons, irritability, difficulty in self-control; pale tongue body, thin and white coating, wiry and thready pulse	Tonify the heart and tranquilize the mind	Classical Formulas: 1. *Gui Pi Tang* Patent Medicines: 1. *Gui Pi Wan* 2. *Suan Zao Ren Tang Wan*	1. *Shen Gem* (HC) 2. *SL-749* (Pro) *Note:* The above can be used in combination.
Deficiency of heart and spleen	Palpitations, timidity, insomnia, forgetfulness, pale complexion, lassitude, dizziness, anorexia; pale tongue body, thready and weak pulse	Invigorate the heart and spleen, tonify qi and blood	Classical Formulas: 1. *Gui Pi Tang* + *Yu Jin, He Huan Hua*	1. Gather Vitality (Jade) + *SL-749* (Pro) 2. *Compassionate Sage* (Jade) 3. *Calm Spirit* (HC) 4. *Shen Gem (HC)*
Yin deficiency	Irritability, impatience, hot temper, dizziness, palpitations, insomnia, nocturnal emission, irregular menstruation, soreness and weakness of the loins and knees; red tongue body, wiry, thready, and rapid pulse	Nourish yin, clear fire, and tranquilize the mind	Classical Formulas: 1. *Liu Wei Di Huang Wan* 2. *Tian Wang Bu Xin Dan* *Note:* The above can be combined to strengthen the effect. 3. *Bai Zi Yang Xin Wan* Patent Medicines: 1. *Liu Wei Di Huang Wan* 2. *Tian Wang Bu Xin Dan* 3. *Bai Zi Yang Xin Wan*	1. *Quiet Contemplative* (Jade) or *Nine Flavor Tea* (HC) + *PM-637* (Pro) 2. *Woman's Balance* (HC) *Note: Celestial Emperor's Blend* (K'an) can be combined with either of the above to strengthen the effect.

PART II

Cross-Reference of Chinese and U.S. Patent Medicines

Key to Label Information

SUPPLIER	ABBREVIATION
Chinese Modular Solution	C
East Tao Herb Pharmacy	E
Five Element Herb Company	F
Golden Flower Chinese Herbs	G
Health Concerns	H
Jade Pharmacy	J
K'an Herbal	K
Long Life Herbal Pharmacy	L
Pro Botanixx	P
Pacific Biologic	PB
The Three Treasures	T
Turtle Mountain	TM

Traditional Formula Pinyin	U.S. Formula English
Ba Wei Di Huang Wan Jia Jian	Rehmannia 8 (H)
Ba Xian Chang Shou Wan	Eight Immortals Formula (G)
Ba Zhen Tang Jia Jian	Women's Precious Formula (G) Eight Treasures (H) Postpartum (H) Women's Precious (J)
Ba Zheng San	Akebia Moist Heat (H) Lower Burner (TM)
Bai He Gu Jin Tang	Lily Preserve Metal Formula (G)

Traditional Formula Pinyin	U.S. Formula English
Bai Hu Tang Jia Jian	Clear Lustre (T)
Bai Tou Weng Tang Jia Jian	Phellostatin (H) Formula H (H)
Bai Zi Yang Xin Wan	Clear the Soul (T)
Ban Xia Bai Zhu Tian Ma Tang	Clear Yang (T)
Ban Xia Hou Po Tang	Open the Heart (T) Pinellia and Magnolia Bark Formula (G)
Bao He Wan	Morning Glory (E)
Bei Xie Fen Qing Yin	Separate Clear and Turbid (T)
Bu Zhong Yi Qi Tang	Ginseng and Astragalus Formula (G) Tonify Qi and Ease the Muscle (T) Arouse Vigor (J) (K) Energy K (E)
Cai Feng Zhen Zhu An Chuang Wan	Colorful Phoenix Pearl Combo (K)
Cang Er Zi San Jia Jian	Welcome Fragrance (T) Xanthium Relieve (H) X Plus (E)
Chai Hu Gui Zhi Tang	Ease 2 (H)
Chai Hu Mu Li Long Gu Tang	Bupleurum D Formula (G) Ease Plus (H)
Chai Hu Shu Gan San	Liver Qi Pacifier (L) Chai Hu Shu Gan San (E)
Chai Hu Xiang Fu Tang	Bupleurum Entangled Qi (H)
Chuan Bei Ban Xia Gao	Fritillaria and Pinellia Syrup (G)
Chuan Xin Lian Kang Yan Pian	Clear Heat (H)

Traditional Formula Pinyin	U.S. Formula English
Da Bu Yin Won Jia Jian	R Plus (E)
Da Huo Luo Dan	*AC-Q* (H)
Dan Shen Jia Si Jun Zi Pian	Salvia Ten Formula (G)
Dan Zhi Xiao Yao San	Smooth Passage (T) Xiao Yao San Plus (L) Woman's Balance (H)
Dan Gui Bu Xue Tan Jia Jian	Radio-Support (T)
Dang Gui Shao Yao San	Tang Kuei and Peony Formula (G)
Di Ding Qing Huo Pian	Viola Clear Fire Formula (G)
Die Da Wan	Tieh Ta Formula (G)
Ding Chuan Wan Jia Jian	Clear Air (H) Asthma AS-135-Cold (P) Asthma AS-137-Heat (P)
Ding Xin Wan	Calm Spirit (H)
Du Huo Ji Sheng Tang	Du Huo and Loranthus Formula (G) Meridian Circulation (J) (K)
Er Chen Tang	Limpid Sea (T) Lucid Clarity (J) (K) PhL-I (E)
Er Xian Tang Jia Jian	Two Immortals (H) Women's Journey (J) Er Xian Tang Plus (E)
Fang Feng Tong Sheng San Jia Jian	Astra 18 Diet (H) Flavor 21 Capsules (E)
Fu Fang Tu Fu Ling Tang	Smilax Compound (E)

Traditional Formula Pinyin	U.S. Formula English
Fu Ling Xiao Hui Xiang Fang	Poria and Fennel Formula (G)
Gan Lu Xiao Du Dan Jia Jian	A.V.D. (E)
Ge Gen Tang	Pueraria Formula (G)
Ge Xia Zhu Yu Tang	Stir Field of Elixir (T)
Gui Pi Tang	Calm the Spirit (T) Shen Gem (H) Gather Vitality (J) (K) Energy A (E)
Gui Zhi Fu Ling Wan	Cinnamon and Poria Formula (G) Women's Palace (J)
Hu Po Yang Xin Dan	Compassionate Sage (J) (K)
Huai Hua San	D.U. Compound (E)
Huang Lian Jie Du Pian	Coptis Relieve Toxicity Formula (G) Q.B.S. (E)
Huang Qi Dong Qing Pian	Astragalus and Ligustrum Formula (G)
Huang Qi Jian Zhong Tang	Astragalus Formula (G)
Huo Luo Xiao Ling Dan	Channel Flow (H)
Huo Po Xia Ling Tang	Drain Fields (T)
Huo Xiang Zheng Qi San	Prime Relief (J) Upper Burner (TM) Early Comfort (K)
Jing Gui Shen Qi Wan Jia Jian	Essential Yang Formula (G) Dynamic Warrior (J) (K)
Jing Huang San	Golden Balm (E)

Traditional Formula Pinyin	U.S. Formula English
Jing Fang Bai Du San	Expel Wind-Cold (G) Prime Rescue (J) Dispel Invasion (K)
Jing Qi Pian	Jing Qi Formula (G)
Jiu Wei Qiang Huo Tang	Head Q (H)
Juan Bi Tang	Juan Bi Formula (G) Brocade Sinews (T) Arthritis AR 125 Shi (p) Arthritis AR 127 XU (p)
Kang Guo Min Wan	Allergease (L)
Kang Ning Wan	Quiet Digestion (H)
Lian Po Yin	Ease the Muscle (T)
Liu Jun Zi Tang Jia Jian	Chemo-Support (T) Six Gentlemen Formula (G) Prosperous Farmer (J) (K)
Liu Wei Di Huang Wan	Nourish Essence Formula (G) Quiet Contemplative (J) (K)
Long Dan Xie Gan Tang Jia Jian	Drain Fire (T) Gentiana Drain Fire Formula (G) Peaceful Sunset (T) Coptis Purge Fire (H) Quell Fire (J) (K) R.D.Y. (E) Gentiana Compound (E)
Ma Huang Tang Jia Jian	Common Cold CO-195 (P)
Ming Mu Di Huang Wan	Ming Mu Formula (G)
Pao Zhen Gao	Herpecream (L)

Traditional Formula Pinyin	U.S. Formula English
Pi Yan Jing	Skin-Cleanser (L)
Ping Wei San Jia Jian	Stomach Tabs (H) Ping Wei San Plus (E)
Qi Hai Yao Fang	Sea of Qi Formula (G)
Qi Ju Di Huang Wan	Wolfberry Compound (E)
Qi Li San	Reinstall K (H)
Qing Huo Shen Shi Tang Jia Jian	R.D.A. (E)
Qing Liang San	Mountain Sophora (E)
Qing Yi Tang Jia Jian	A.V.B. (E)
Ren Shen Ge Jie San	Ginseng and Gecko (H)
Ren Shen Yang Ying Wan	Ginseng Nourishing Formula (G)
Run Chang Wan	Smooth Response (K)
San Qi Pian	San Qi Formula (G)
Sha Shen Mai Dong Tang Jia Jian	Herbal Sentinel Yin (T) Jade Spring (T) Wise Judge (J)
Shao Yao Gan Cao Jia Yan Hu Tang	Corydalis Formula (G) Lily 14 (BP)
She Chuang Zi San Jia Jian	Lotus Balm (E)
Shen Ling Bai Zhu San Jia Jian	Central Mansion (T) Middle Burner (TM) Cleansing Formula (E)

Traditional Formula Pinyin	U.S. Formula English
Shen Rong Wan Jia Jian	Tian Jui T-M (E)
Shen Tong Zhu Yu Tang Jia Jian	Meridian Passage (J) (K)
Sheng Hua Tang	Uterus-A (L)
Sheng Mai San Jia Jian	Sheng Mai San Plus (E)
Shi Quan Da Bu Wan	General Tonic Formula (G)
Shi Wu Wei Fu Ling Pian	Poria 15 Formula (G)
Shou Wu Pian	He Shou Wu Tablets (G)
Shu Jing Huo Xue Tang	Clematis and Stephania Formula (G) Mobility 2 (H)
Si Jun Zi Tang Jia Jian	Astra 8 (H)
Si Mao Wan	Si Mao San (L)
Si Wu Tang Jia Wei	Bend Bamboo (T) Tang Kuei and Salvia Formula (G) Women's Rhythm (J) Q.B.R. (E) Tian Kui T-F (E)
Su He Xiang Tang Jia Jian	Cir-Q (H)
Su Zi Jiang Qi Tang	Clear Qi (T)
Suan Zao Ren Tang	Zizyphus Formula (G)
Suo Quan Wan Jia Jian	Restore Integrity (K)
Tian Ma Gou Teng Yin	Gastrodia and Uncaria Formula (G) Gastrodia Relieve Wind (H) G Plus (E)

Traditional Formula Pinyin	U.S. Formula English
Tian Wang Bu Xin Dan	Heavenly Emperor's Formula (G) Energy S (E) Celestial Emperor's Blend (K)
Tong Jing Wan	Crampbark Plus (H)
Tong Luo San	Blood Circulation BC-147 (P)
Wan Dai Tang Jia Jian	Golden Rose (E)
Wan Du Hua Yu Tang	Backbone (H)
Wen Dan Tang	Clear Phlegm (H)
Wu Hua Tang	Wu Hua Formula (G)
Wu Jia Shen Pian	Siberian Ginseng Tablets (G)
Wu Ling San Jia Jian	Drain Dampness (H) Ling Syndrome Formula (E) Water's Way (K)
Wu Mei Wan	Wu Mei Wan Plus (E)
Wu Wei Xiao Du Yin	Five Detox (L)
Xiang Sha Liu Jun Zi Tang	Soothe the Center Six Gentlemen (H)
Xiao Chai Hu Tang Jia Jian	Minor Bupleurum formula (G) Shaoyang Formula (E)
Xiao Nei Wan Jia Jian	Q.B.H. (E)
Xiao Qing Long Tang	Minor Bluegreen Dragon Formula (G) Minor Blue Dragon (H)
Xiao Yao San	Bupleurum and Tang Kuei Formula (G) Freeing the Moon (T) Relaxed Wanderer (J) (K)

Traditional Formula Pinyin	U.S. Formula English
Xiao Yao San Jia Wei	Break into a Smile (T) Free and Easy Wanderer Plus (G) Energy E (E) Green Xiao Yao San (E) Shu Xie Tea (E) Women's Relaxing (E) Yellow Xiao Yao San (E)
Xue Fu Zhu Yu Tanag	Red Stirring (T) Q.B.A. (E)
Yang Xin Ning Shen Wan	Peaceful Spirit Formula (G)
Yang Yin Qing Fei Tang Jia Jian	Energy C (E)
Yi Guan Jian Jia Jian	Fertile Garden (H) Q.B.Y. (E)
Yi Min Tang	Allergy AL-113 (P)
Yin Qiao San Jia Jian	Expel Wind-Heat (T) Yin Chiao Formula (G) Prime Response (J) Cold and Flue CO-197 (P) A.V.A. (E) B Plus (E) Light Clearing (E) Yin Qiao (K) Initial Defense (K)
You Gui Wan Jia Jian	Ease the Journey—Yang (T) Strengthen the Root (T) Energy D (E)

Traditional Formula Pinyin	U.S. Formula English
Yu Die Wan	Pang Da Hai Compound (E)
Yu Ping Feng Jia Jian	Herbal Sentinel—Yang (T) Jade Screen and Xanthium formula (G) Jade Screen (T) Astra C (H) Jade Screen (E)
Zhi Bai Di Huang Wan Jia Jian	Clear the Root (T) Rehmannia and Scrophularia Formula (G) Nine Flavor Tea (H) Temper Fire (J)
Zhong Gan Ling Pian	Zhong Gan Ling Formula (G)
Zhui Feng Tou Gu Wan	Chase Wind, Penetrate Bone Formula (G)
Zi Cao Quai Ban Tang	Zi Cao Compound (E)
Zuo Gui Wan Ji Jian	Ease the Journey—Yin (T) Nourish the Root (T) True Yin formula (G) Astra Essence (H) Energy L (E)

PART III

U.S. Formula Ingredients List

China Herb Company

Clear Lungs

INGREDIENTS

Radix Platycodi Grandiflora	Jie geng	桔 梗
Tuber Ophiopogonis Japonici	Mai men dong	麥 門 冬
Rhizoma Belamcamdae Chinensis	She gan	射 干
Semen Trichosanthis Kirilowii	Gua lou ren	瓜 蔞 仁
Fructus Arctii Lappae	Niu bang zi	牛 蒡 子
Radix Isatidis seu Baphicacanthi	Ban lan gen	板 蘭 根
Radix Angelicae Dahuricae	Bai zhi	白 芷
Radix Achyranthis Aspera	Dao kou cao	倒 扣 草
Flos Magnoliae liliflor	Xin yi hua	辛 荑 花
Radix Glycyrrhizae Uralensis	Gan cao	甘 草
Herba Menthae	Bo he	薄 荷
Fennel	Xiao Hui Xiang	小 茴 香

Clear Skin

INGREDIENTS

Radix Bupleuri	Chai hu	柴 胡
Radix Angelicae Dahuricae	Bai zhi	白 芷
Ramulus Loranthi seu Visci	Sang ji sheng	桑 寄 生
Herba Hedyotidis Diffusae	Bai hua she she cao	白 花 蛇 舌 草
Radix Astragali	Huang qi	黃 耆
Spica Prunellae Vulgaris	Xia ku cao	夏 枯 草
Radix Saussureae seu Vladimiriae	Mu xiang	木 香
Herba Taraxaci Mongolici cum Radice	Pu gong ying	蒲 公 英
Rhizoma Zingiberis Officinalis	Gan jiang	乾 姜
Radix Sophorae Flavescentis	Ku shen	苦 參
Radix Rehmannai	Di huang	地 黃

Clear Vision

INGREDIENTS

Nlss Digestible spirulina/chlorella		
Fructus Lycii Chinensis	Gou qi zi	枸 杞 子
Flos Chrysanthemi Morifolii	Ju hua	菊 花
Radix Ginseng	Ren shen	人 參
Radix Polygoni Multiflori	Shou wu	首 烏
Frutus Ligustri Lucidi	Nu zhen zi	女 貞 子
Spica Prunellae Vulgaris	Xia ku cao	夏 枯 草
Buddliea Officinalis	Mi meng hua	密 蒙 花
Semen Cassia Tarae	Jue ming zi	决 明 子
Rhizoma Zingiberis Officinalis	Gan jiang	乾 姜
Rhizoma Acori Graminei	Shi chang pu	石 菖 莆
Folium Ginkgo Bilobae	Bai guo ye	白 果 葉

Detox Compound

INGREDIENTS

Spica Prunellae Vulgaris	Xia ku cao	夏 枯 草
Rhizoma Coptidis	Huang lian	黄 連
Radix Scutellariae Baicalensis	Huang qin	黄 芩
Radix Isatidis seu Baphicacanthi	Ban lan gen	板 蘭 根
Myrrha Mo yao	Mo yao	沒 藥
Herba Hedyotidis Diffusae	Bai hua she she cao	白 花 蛇 舌 草
Radix Bupleuri	Chai hu	柴 胡
Semen Sterculiae Scaphigerae	Pang da hai	胖 大 海
Rhizoma Zingiberis Officinalis	Gan jiang	乾 姜
Herba Taraxaci Mongolici cum Radice	Pu gong ying	蒲 公 英
Red Clover Blossom		
Burdock root		
Goldenseal root		
Nlss Digestible spirulina/chlorella		
Echinacea purpura		

Ear Clear

INGREDIENTS

Radix Bupleuri	Chai hu	柴 胡
Flos Lonicerae Japonicae	Yin hua	銀 花
Semen Coicis	Yi yi ren	薏 苡 仁
Rhizoma Pinelliae Ternatae	Fa ban xia	法 半 夏
Rhizoma Acori Graminei	Shi chang pu	石 菖 蒲
Rhizoma Atractylodis Macrocephalae	Bai zhu	白 朮
Pericarpium Citri Reticulatae	Chen pi	陳 皮
Ramulus Cinnamomi Cassiae	Gui zhi	桂 枝
Radix Paeoniae Lactiflorae	Bai shao	白 芍
Radix Glycyrrhizae Uralensis	Gan cao	甘 草
Rhizoma Zingiberis Officialis Recens	Sheng jiang	生 姜
Fructus Zizyphi Jujubae	Da zao	大 棗
Maltose		

Full Circle

INGREDIENTS

Nlss Digestible spirulina/chlorella		
Herba Cistanches	Rou cong rong	肉 蓯 蓉
Herba Epimedii	Yin yang huo	淫 羊 藿
Radix Angelicae Sinensis	Dang gui	當 歸
Radix Rehmanniae Glutinosae Conquitae	Shu di huang	熟 地 黃
Radix Paeoniae Lactiflorae	Bai shao	白 芍
Cacumen Biotae Orientalis	Ce bai ye	側 柏 葉
Fructus Zizyphi Jujubae	Da zao	大 棗
Cortex Albizziae Julibrissin	He huan pi	合 歡 皮
Radix Anemarrhenae	Zhi mu	知 母
Cortex Phellodendri	Huang bai	黃 柏
Radix Glycyrrhizae Uralensis	Gan cao	甘 草
Royal jelly		
Vitamin E		

Invigorate QB

INGREDIENTS

Rhizoma Cyperi Rotudi	Xiang fu	香 附
Rhizoma Corydalis	Yan hu suo	延 胡 索
Radix Paeoniae Lactiflorae	Bai shao	白 芍
Radix Bupleuri	Chai hu	柴 胡
Pericarpium Citri Reticulatae	Chen pi	陳 皮
Fructus Immaturus Citri Aurantii	Zhi shi	枳 實
Pericarpium Citri Reticulatae Viride	Qing pi	青 皮
Radix Linderae Strychnifoliae	Wu yao	烏 藥
Cortex Magnoliae Offcinalis	Hou po	厚 樸
Lignum Aquilariae	Chen xiang	沉 香
Arillus Euphoriae Longanae	Long yan rou	龍 眼 肉
Radix Glycyrrhizae Uralensis	Gan cao	甘 草
Fructus Amomi	Sha ren	砂 仁
Radix Salviae Miltiorrhizae	Dan shen	丹 參
Radix Ligustici Wallichii	Chuan xiong	川 芎
Leonori		

Prostate Combination

INGREDIENTS

Saw palmetto fruit concentrate		
Radix Achyranthis Bidentatae	Niu xi	牛 膝
Semen Plantaginis	Che qian zi	車 前 子
Semen Vaccariae Segetalis	Wang bu liu xing	王 不 留 行
Extremitas Radicis Angelicae Sinensis	Dang gui wei	當 歸 尾
Radix Paeoniae Rubrae	Chi shao	赤 芍
Cortex Moutan Radicis	Mu dan pi	牡 丹 皮
Radix Ginseng	Ren shen	人 參
Radix Linderae Strychnifoliae	Wu yao	烏 藥
Rhizoma Zingiberis Officialis Recens	Sheng jiang	生 姜
Fennel		
Vitamin B6		
Zinc Picolinate		

Smooth Cycle

INGREDIENTS

Nlss Digestible spirulina/chlorella		
Radix Angelicae Sinensis	Dang gui	當 歸
Rhizoma Corydalis	Yan hu suo	延 胡 索
Rhizoma Cyperi Rotudi	Xiang fu	香 附
Radix Saussureae seu Vladimiriae	Mu xiang	木 香
Radix Linderae Strychnifoliae	Wu yao	烏 藥
Radix et Caulis Jixueteng	Ji xue teng	雞 血 藤
Fructus seu Semen Amomi	Sha ren	砂 仁
Herba Leonuri Heterophylli	Yi mu cao	益 母 草
Radix Paeoniae Lactiflorae	Bai shao	白 芍
Cortex Albizziae Julibrissin	He huan pi	合 歡 皮
Radix Bupleuri	Chai hu	柴 胡
Radix Glycyrrhizae Uralensis	Gan cao	甘 草

Chinese Modular Solutions

Chest Relief

INGREDIENTS

Bulbus Fritillariae Thunbergii	Zhe bei mu	浙 貝 母
Radix Platycodi Grandiflori	Jie geng	桔 梗
Concretio Silicea Bambusae	Tian zhu huang	天 竹 黃
Radix Scorphulariae Ning poensis	Xuan shen	玄 參
Radix Scutellariae Baicalensis	Huang qin	黃 芩
Radix Stemonae	Zhi bai bu	制 百 部
Percarpium citri Reticulatae	Chen pi	陳 皮
Sclerotium Poriae Cocos	Fu ling	茯 苓
Redix Glycyrrhizae Uralensis	Gan cao	甘 草
Rhizoma Zingiberis Officinalis	Gan jiang	乾 姜
Semen Trichosanthis Kirilowii	Gua lou ren	瓜 蔞 仁
Folium Mori Albae	Sang ye	桑 葉

INGREDIENTS CONTINUED FROM PAGE 117

Radix Pseudostellariae Heterophyllae	Tai zi shen	太子參
Frutus Schisandrae Chinensis	Wu wei zi	五味子
Rhizoma Polygonati Odorati	Yu zhu	玉竹
Fructus Immaturus Citri Aurantii	Zhi shi	枳實
Semen Perillae	Zi su zi	紫蘇子
Cortex Magnoliae Officinalis	Hou po	厚樸
Radix Polygale Tenuifoliae Recens	Yuan zhi	遠志
Radix Paeoniae Lactiflorae	Bai shao	白芍

Cluster Dissolving

INGREDIENTS

Herba Hedyotidis Diffusae	Bai hua she she cao	白花蛇舌草
Herba Scutellariae Barbatae	Ban zhi lian	半枝蓮
Herba Selaginellae Doederleinii	Shi shang bai	石上白
Rhizoma Atractylodis Macrocephalae	Bai zhu	白朮
Herba Taraxaci Mongolici cum Radice	Pu gong ying	蒲公英
Radix Sophorae Tonkinensis	Shan dou gen	山豆根
Radix Sophorae Flavescentis	Ku shen	苦參
Radix Isatidis seu Baphicacanthi	Ban lan gen	板蘭根
Zanthoxylum Nitidum	Liang main zhen	兩面針
Rhizoma Curcumae Zedoariae	E zhu	莪朮
Rhizoma Sparganii	San leng	三稜

Consolidate Qi

INGREDIENTS

Radix Astragali	Huang qi	黃耆
Radix Dioscoreae Oppositae	Shan yao	山藥
Semen Nelumbins	Lian zi	蓮子
Semen Euryales Ferocis	Qian shi	芡實
Semen Myristicae Fragrantis	Rou dou kou	肉豆蔻
Rhizoma Atractylodis Macrocephalae	Bai zhu	白朮
Radix Ledebouriellae Sesloidis	Fang feng	防風

Comfort Shen

INGREDIENTS

Concha Margaritifera	Zhen zhu mu	珍 珠 母
Sclerotium Poriae Cocos Paradicis	Fu shen	茯 神
Os Draconis	Long gu	龍 骨
Calcined Magnetite	Ci shi	磁 石
Radix Polygale Tenuifoliae Recens	Yuan zhi	遠 志
Ganoderma Japonicum	Ling zhi	靈 芝
Caulis Polygoni Multiflori	Ye jiao teng	夜 交 藤
Tuber Ophiopogonis Japonici	Mai men dong	麥 門 冬
Semen Zizyphi Spinosae	Suan zao ren	酸 棗 仁
Radix Ligustici Wallichii	Chuan xiong	川 芎
Succinum	Hu po	琥 珀
Frutus Schisandrae Chinensis	Wu wei zi	五 味 子

Disperse Qi

INGREDIENTS

Fructus Hordei Vulgaris Germinantus	Mai Ya	麥 芽
Radix Saussureae seu Vladimiriae	Mu xiang	木 香
Rhizoma Cyperi Rotundi	Xiang fu	香 附
Percarpium citri Reticulatae	Chen pi	陳 皮
Pericarpium Citri Reticulatae Viride	Qing pi	青 皮
Fructus Citri Aurantii	Zhi ke	枳 殼
Cortex Magnoliae Officinalis	Hou po	厚 樸
Fructus seu Semen Amomi	Sha ren	砂 仁
Semen Perillae	Zi su zi	紫 蘇 子
Radix Platycodi Grandiflori	Jie geng	桔 梗
Rhizoma Coptidis	Huang lian	黃 連

Disperse Moisture

INGREDIENTS

Semen Coicis	Yi yi ren	薏 苡 仁
Sclerotium Poriae Cocos	Fu ling	茯 苓
Semen Arecae Catechu	Bing lang	檳 榔
Rhizoma Alismatis Plantago-aquaticae	Ze xie	澤 瀉
Rhizoma Dioscoreae Hypogloaucae	Bei xie	萆 薢
Rhizoma Pinelliae Ternatae	Fa ban xia	法 半 夏
Herba Angastache seu Pogostemi	Huo xiang	藿 香
Radix Saussureae seu Vladimiriae	Mu xiang	木 香
Rhizoma Atractyloidis	Cang zhu	蒼 朮

Disperse Blood

INGREDIENTS

Radix Salviae	Dan shen	丹 參
Fasciculus Vascularis Luffae	Si gua luo	絲 瓜 絡
Radix Paeoniae Lactiflorae	Bai shao	白 芍
Herba Lycopi Lucidi	Ze lan	澤 蘭
Tuber Curcumae	Yu jin	郁 金
Radix Ligustici Wallichii	Chuan xiong	川 芎
Herba Artemisiae Anomalae	Liu ji nu	劉 寄 奴
Fructus Immaturus Citri Aurantii	Zhi shi	枳 實
Rhizoma Cyperi Rotundi	Xiang fu	香 附
Ramulus Cinnamomi	Gui zhi	桂 枝

Ease Strain

INGREDIENTS

St. John's Wort concentrate		
Pulvis Arisaemae cum Felle Bovis	Dan nan xing	膽 南 星
Roasted Rhizoma Typhonii Gigantei	Zhi bai fu zi	制 白 附 子
Ramulus Uncariae	Gou teng	鉤 藤
Cormu Antelopis	Ling yang jiao	羚 羊 角
Os Draconis	Long gu	龍 骨
Rhizoma Acori Graminei	Shi chang pu	石 菖 蒲
Radix Polygale Tenuifoliae Recens	Yuan zhi	遠 志
Cortex Albizziae Julibrissin	He huan pi	合 歡 皮
Semen Zizyphi Spinosae	Suan zao ren	酸 棗 仁
Caulis Polygoni Multiflori	Ye jiao teng	夜 交 藤
Rhizoma Pinelliae Ternatae	Fa ban xia	法 半 夏
Bulbus Fritillariae	Chuan bei mu	川 貝 母
Radix Paeoniae Lactiflorae	Bai shao	白 芍
Flos Chrysanthemi Morifolii	Bai ju hua	白 菊 花
Fructus Gardiniae Jasminoidis	Shan zhi zi	山 梔 子
Radix Bupleuri	Chai hu	柴 胡
Radix Peucedaani	Qian hu	前 胡
Fructus Immaturus Citri Aurantii	Zhi shi	枳 實
Radix Ligustici Wallichii	Chuan xiong	川 芎
Bulbus Lilii	Bai he	百 合
Tuber Ophiopogonis Japonici	Mai men dong	麥 門 冬
Succinum	Hu po	琥 珀

Harmonize Heart and Lung

INGREDIENTS

Ilex Pubescens Hook. Et Arn	Mao dong qing	毛冬青
Bulbus Lilii	Bai he	百合
Radix Scutellariae Baicalensis	Huang qin	黄芩
Sclerotium Ganodermae	Ling zhi cao	靈芝草
Bulbus Fritillariae Thunbergii	Zhe bei mu	浙貝母
Radix Platycodi Grandiflori	Jie geng	桔梗
Radix Polygale Tenuifoliae Recens	Yuan zhi	遠志
Calcined Magnetite	Ci shi	磁石
Sclerotium Poriae Cocos Pararadicis	Fu shen	茯神
Redix Glycyrrhizae Uralensis	Gan cao	甘草
Rhizoma Pinelliae Ternatae	Fa ban xia	法半夏
Semen Trichosanthis Kirilowii	Gua lou ren	瓜蔞仁
Frutus Schisandrae Chinensis	Wu wei zi	五味子

Harmonize Kidney and Heart

INGREDIENTS

Radix Rehmanniae Glutinosae Conquitae	Shu di huang	熟地黄
Radix Salviae Miltiorrhizae	Dan shen	丹參
Radix Polygale Tenuifoliae Recens	Yuan zhi	遠志
Ganoderma Japonicum	Ling zhi	靈芝
Frutus Schisandrae Chinensis	Wu wei zi	五味子
Semen Nelumbins	Lian zi	蓮子
Radix Anemarrhenae	Zhi mu	知母
Rhizoma Coptidis	Huang lian	黄連
Fructus seu Semen Amomi	Sha ren	砂仁
Herba Leonuri Heterophylli	Yi mu cao	益母草
Os Draconis	Long gu	龍骨
Caulis Polygoni Multiflori	Ye jiao teng	夜交藤
Lignum Aquilariae	Chen xiang	沉香
Redix Glycyrrhizae Uralensis	Gan cao	甘草

Harmonize Liver and Spleen

INGREDIENTS

Radix Bupleuri	Chai hu	柴 胡
Rhizoma Cyperi Rotundi	Xiang fu	香 附
Radix Saussureae seu Vladimiriae	Mu xiang	木 香
Rhizoma Atractylodis Macrocephalae	Bai zhu	白 朮
Sclerotium Poriae Cocos	Fu ling	茯 苓
Radix Ledebouriellae Sesloidis	Fang feng	防 風
Radix Paeoniae Lactiflorae	Bai shao	白 芍
Fructus Immaturus Citri Aurantii	Zhi shi	枳 實
Pericarpium Citri Reticulatae Viride	Qing pi	青 皮
Radix Angelicae Sinensis	Dang gui	當 歸
Herba Menthae	Bo he	薄 荷
Fructus Crataegi roasted	Shan zha jiao	山 楂 焦
Redix Glycyrrhizae Uralensis	Gan cao	甘 草

Harmonize Spleen and Kidney

INGREDIENTS

Sclerotium Poriae Cocos	Fu ling	茯 苓
Sclerotium Polypori Umbellati	Zhu ling	豬 苓
Rhizoma Atractylodis Macrocephalae	Bai zhu	白 朮
Rhizoma Alismatis Plantago-aquaticae	Ze xie	澤 瀉
Radix Astragali	Huang qi	黃 耆
Percarpium citri Reticulatae	Chen pi	陳 皮
Fructus Citri Aurantii	Zhi ke	枳 殼
Semen Arecae Catechu	Bing lang	檳 榔
Semen Euryales Ferocis	Qian shi	芡 實
Redix Glycyrrhizae Uralensis	Gan cao	甘 草
Radix Ledebouriellae Sesloidis	Fang feng	防 風

Meal Mover

INGREDIENTS

Fructus Crataegi roasted	Shan zha jiao	山 楂 焦
Massa Fermentata	Shen qu	神 曲
Radix Saussureae seu Vladimiriae	Mu xiang	木 香
Semen Arecae Catechu	Bing lang	檳 榔
Sclerotium Poriae	Cocos Fu ling	茯 苓
Fructus Forsythiae SuspensaeLian qiao	Lian qiao	連 翹
Percarpium citri Reticulatae	Chen pi	陳 皮
Radix et Rhizoma Rhei	Da huang	大 黄
Rhizoma Pinelliae Ternatae	Fa ban xia	法 半 夏
Semen Paphani Sativi	Lai fu zi	萊 菔 子
Fructus seu Semen Amomi	Sha ren	砂 仁

Move Mountains

INGREDIENTS

Radix Ginseng	Ji lin shen	吉 林 參
Radix Astragali	Huang qi	黄 耆
Frutus Schisandrae Chinensis	Wu wei zi	五 味 子
Frutus Lycii Chinensis	Gou qi zi	枸 杞 子
Herba Dendrobii	Shi hu	石 斛
Phlogisticlean		

Philogisticlean

INGREDIENTS

Radix Isatidis seu Baphicacanthi	Ban lan gen	板 蘭 根
Fructificatio Lasiosphaerae seu Calvatiae	Ma bo	馬 勃
Radix Scorphulariae Ning poensis	Xuan shen	玄 參
Herba Hedyotidis Diffusae	Bai hua she she cao	白 花 蛇 舌 草
Cortex Moutan Radicis	Mu dan pi	牡 丹 皮
Cortex Phellodendri	Huang bai	黄 柏

Purge Qi

INGREDIENTS

Semen Paphani Sativi	Lai fu zi	萊菔子
Fructus Crataegi roasted	Shan zha jiao	山楂焦
Radix Saussureae seu Vladimiriae	Mu xiang	木香
Rhizoma Cyperi Rotundi	Xiang fu	香附
Semen Perillae	Zi su zi	紫蘇子
Cortex Magnoliae Officinalis	Hou po	厚樸
Semen Arecae Catechu	Bing lang	檳榔
Rhizoma Coptidis	Huang lian	黃連
Radix et Rhizoma Rhei	Da huang	大黃
Redix Glycyrrhizae Uralensis	Gan cao	甘草
Fructus Citri Aurantii	Zhi ke	枳殼
Fructus Immaturus Citri Aurantii	Zhi shi	枳實

Purge Blood

INGREDIENTS

Ilex Pubescens Hook. Et Arn	Mao dong qing	毛冬青
Herba Leonuri Heterophylli	Yi mu cao	益母草
Radix Salviae Miltiorrhizae	Dan shen	丹參
Flos Carthami Tinctorii	Hong hua	紅花
Rhizoma Corydalis Yanhusua	Yan hu suo	延胡索
Herba Lycopi Lucidi	Ze lan	澤蘭
Radix Achyranthis Bidentatae	Huai niu xi	淮牛膝
Radix Paeoniae Rubrae	Chi shao	赤芍
Radix Ligustici Wallichii	Chuan xiong	川芎
Rhizoma Cyperi Rotundi	Xiang fu	香附
Rhizoma Curcumae zedoariae	E zhu	莪朮
Rhizoma Sparganii	San leng	三稜
Semen Vaccariae Segetalis	Wang bu liu xing	王不留行
Sanguis Draconis	Xue jie	血竭

Purge Cold

INGREDIENTS

Semen Trigonellae Foeni-fraeci	Hu lu ba	胡 蘆 巴
Semen Psoraleae Corylifoliae	Bu gu zhi	補 骨 脂
Ramulus Cinnamomi	Gui zhi	桂 枝
Radix Glycyrrhizae Uralensis	Zhi gan cao	炙 甘 草
Rhizoma Zingiberis Officinalis	Gan jiang	乾 姜
Fructus Piperis Longi	Bi ba	蓽 拔
Fructus Evodiae	Wu zhu yu	吳 茱 萸
Radix Aconiti Carmichaelai Praeparata	Fu zi	附 子

Purge Heat

INGREDIENTS

Flos Lonicerae Japonicae	Jin yin hua	金 銀 花
Fructus Forsythiae Suspensae	Lian qiao	連 翹
Flos Chrysanthemi Indici	Ye ju hua	野 菊 花
Spica Prunellae Vulgaris	Xia ku cao	夏 枯 草
Gypsum	Shi gao	石 膏
Herba Andrographitis Paniculatae	Chuan xin lian	穿 心 蓮
Herba Taraxaci Mongolici cum Radice	Pu gong ying	蒲 公 英
Radix Scutellariae Baicalensis	Huang qin	黃 芩
Radix Anemarrhenae	Zhi mu	知 母
Radix Rehmanniae	Sheng di huang	生 地 黃
Radix Bupleuri	Chai hu	柴 胡
Redix Glycyrrhizae Uralensis	Gan cao	甘 草

Purge Damp Heat

INGREDIENTS

Sclerotium Poriae Cocos	Fu ling	茯 苓
Rhizoma Alismatis Plantago-aquaticae	Ze xie	澤 瀉
Semen Plantaginis	Che qian zi	車 前 子
Herba Artemisiae Yinchenhao	Yin chen hao	茵 陳 蒿
Fructus Immaturus Citri Aurantii	Zhi shi	枳 實
Caulis Mutong	Mu tong	木 通
Radix Scutellariae Baicalensis	Huang qin	黃 芩
Fructus Gardeniae	Zhi zi	梔 子
Herba Andrographitis Paniculatae	Chuan xin lian	穿 心 蓮
Radix Sophorae Flavescentis	Ku shen	苦 參
Fructus Forsythiae Suspensae	Lian qiao	連 翹
Redix Glycyrrhizae Uralensis	Gan cao	甘 草
Fructus Evodiae	Wu zhu yu	吳 茱 萸

Purge Phlegm

INGREDIENTS

Sclerotium Poriae Cocos	Fu ling	茯 苓
Herba Sargassii	Hai zao	海 藻
Bulbus Fritillariae Thunbergii	Zhe bei mu	浙 貝 母
Radix Stemonae	Zhi bai bu	制 百 部
Semen Trichosanthis Kirilowii	Gua lou ren	瓜 蔞 仁
Radix Platycodi Grandiflori	Jie geng	桔 梗
Rhizoma Pinelliae Ternatae	Fa ban xia	法 半 夏
Pulvis Arisaemae cum Felle Bovis	Dan nan xing	膽 南 星
Semen Perillae	Zi su zi	紫 蘇 子
Concretio Silicea Bambusae	Tian zhu huang	天 竹 黃
Percarpium citri Reticulatae	Chen pi	陳 皮
Fructus Immaturus Citri Aurantii	Zhi shi	枳 實
Cortex Magnoliae Officinalis	Hou po	厚 樸

Purge Internal Wind

INGREDIENTS

Rhizoma Gastrodiae Elatae	Tian ma	天 麻
Ramulus Uncariae	Gou teng	鉤 藤
Radix Paeoniae Lactiflorae	Bai shao	白 芍
Ramus Loranthi seu Visci	Sang ji sheng	桑 寄 生
Concha Haliotidis	Shi jue ming	石 決 明
Flos Chrysanthemi Morifolii	Huang ju hua	黃 菊 花
Fructus Tribuli Terrestris	Bai ji li	白 蒺 藜
Flos Chrysanthemi Morifolii	Bai ju hua	白 菊 花
Semen Cassia Tarae	Jue ming zi	決 明 子
Ramulus Mori Albae	Sang zhi	桑 枝
Frutus Mori Albae	Sang shen	桑 椹

Purge External Wind

INGREDIENTS

Radix Puerariae	Ge gen	葛 根
Radix Ledebouriellae Sesloidis	Fang feng	防 風
Rhizoma et Radix Notopterygii	Qiang huo	羌 活
Radix Angelicae	Bai zhi	白 芷
Radix Bupleuri	Chai hu	柴 胡
Radix Ligustici Wallichii	Chuan xiong	川 芎
Rhizoma et Radix Ligustici	Gao ben	藁 本
Herba Menthae	Bo he	薄 荷
Herba cum Radice Asari	Xi xin	細 辛
Folium Mori Albae	Sang ye	桑 葉
Flos Magnoliae liliflor	Xin yi hua	辛 夷 花
Flos Chrysanthemi Morifolii	Huang ju hua	黃 菊 花
Redix Glycyrrhizae Uralensis	Gan cao	甘 草

Replinish Essence

INGREDIENTS

Eleutheroginseng	Wu jia shen	五加參
Fructus Lycii	Gou qi zi	枸杞子
Cornu Cervi Degelatinatium	Lu jiao jiao	鹿角膠
Gelatinum Plastri Testudinis	Gui ban jiao	龜板膠
Radix Paeoniae Lactiflorae	Bai shao	白芍
Cortex Eucommiae Ulmoidis	Du zhong	杜仲
Ramus Loranthi seu Visci	Sang ji sheng	桑寄生
Fructus Corni Officinalis	Shan zhu yu	山茱萸
Frutus Schisandrae Chinensis	Wu wei zi	五味子
Herba Epimedii	Yin yang huo	淫羊藿
Semen Cuscutae	Tu si zi	兎絲子
Semen Nelumbinis Nuciferae	Lian xu	蓮須
Fluoritum	Zi shi ying	紫石英
Semen Cuscutae	Tu si zi	兎絲子
Fructus seu Semen Amomi	Sha ren	砂仁
Rhizoma Alismatis Plantago-aquaticae	Ze xie	澤瀉
Placenta Hominis	Zi he che	紫河車
Radix Scutellariae Baicalensis	Huang qin	黃芩
Cortex Phellodendri	Huang bai	黃柏

Resilience

INGREDIENTS

Radix Astragali	Huang qi	黃耆
Sclerotium Ganodermae	Ling zhi	靈芝
Grifola frondosa fungus	maitake	
Sclerotium Polypori Umbellati	Zhu ling	猪苓
Fructificatio tremellae Fuciformis	Bai mu er	白木耳

Strengthen Liver

INGREDIENTS

Radix Rehmanniae Glutinosae Conquitae	Shu di huang	熟地黄
Radix Paeoniae Lactiflorae	Bai shao	白芍
Frutus Lycii Chinensis	Gou qi zi	枸杞子
Semen Zizyphi Spinosae	Suan zao ren	酸棗仁
Radix Bupleuri	Chai hu	柴胡
Flos Chrysanthemi Morifolii	Huang ju hua	黄菊花
Folium Mori Albae	Sang ye	桑葉
Cortex Moutan Radicis	Mu dan pi	牡丹皮
Radix Ligustici Wallichii	Chuan xiong	川芎
Fructus Citri Aurantii	Zhi ke	枳殼
Pericarpium Citri Reticulatae Viride	Qing pi	青皮
Rhizoma Cyperi Rotundi	Xiang fu	香附
Radix Glycyrrhizae Uralensis	Zhi gan cao	炙甘草

Strengthen Heart

INGREDIENTS

Radix Salviae Miltiorrhizae	Dan shen	丹參
Sclerotium Poriae Cocos Pararadicis	Fu shen	茯神
Semen Zizyphi Spinosae	Suan zao ren	酸棗仁
Frutus Schisandrae Chinensis	Wu wei zi	五味子
Herba Lophatheri Gracilis	Dan zhu ye	淡竹葉
Tuber Ophiopogonis Japonici	Mai men dong	麥門冬
Radix Polygale Tenuifoliae Recens	Yuan zhi	遠志
Radix Ginseng	Ji lin shen	吉林參
Semen Nelumbins	Lian zi	蓮子
Plumula Nelumbinis Nuciferae	Lian zi xin	蓮子心
Radix Glycyrrhizae Uralensis	Zhi gan cao	炙甘草

Strengthen Lung

INGREDIENTS

Radix Astragali	Huang qi	黃耆
Bulbus Fritillariae Thunbergii	Zhe bei mu	浙貝母
Frutus Schisandrae Chinensis	Wu wei zi	五味子
Roasted Radix Anemarrhenae	Chao zhi mu	炒知母
Radix Platycodi Grandiflori	Jie geng	桔梗
Semen Perillae	Zi su zi	紫蘇子
Rhizoma Zingiberis Officinalis	Gan jiang	乾姜
Cortex Mori Albae Raicis	Sang bai pi	桑白皮
Folium Mori Albae	Sang ye	桑葉
Percarpium citri Reticulatae	Chen pi	陳皮
Redix Glycyrrhizae Uralensis	Gan cao	甘草

Strengthen Kidney

INGREDIENTS

Radix Dioscoreae Oppositae	Shan yao	山藥
Fructus Corni Officinalis	Shan zhu yu	山茱萸
Sclerotium Poriae Cocos	Fu ling	茯苓
Rhizoma Alismatis Plantago-aquaticae	Ze xie	澤瀉
Radix Rehmanniae Glutinosae Conquitae	Shu di huang	熟地黃
Radix Rehmanniae	Sheng di huang	生地黃
Frutus Schisandrae Chinensis	Wu wei zi	五味子
Semen Cuscutae	Tu si zi	兎絲子
Cortex Eucommiae Ulmoidis	Du zhong	杜仲
Radix Anemarrhenae	Zhi mu	知母
Fructus seu Semen Amomi	Sha ren	砂仁

Tonify Blood

INGREDIENTS

Radix Astragali Membranalis	Huang qi	黄 者
Radix et Caulis Jixueteng	Ji xue teng	雞 血 藤
Radix Rehmanniae Glutinosae Conquitae	Shu di huang	熟 地 黄
Radix Polygoni Multiflori	He shou wu	何 首 烏
Radix Paeoniae Lactiflorae	Bai shao	白 芍
Fructus Crataegi	Shan zha	山 楂
Radix Polygoni Multiflori	Shou wu	首 烏
Radix Angelicae Sinensis	Dang gui	當 歸
Arillus Euphoriae Longanae	Long yan rou	龍 眼 肉

Tonify Moisture

INGREDIENTS

Herba Dendrobii	Shi hu	石 斛
Rhizoma Polygonati Odorati	Yu zhu	玉 竹
Sclerotium Poriae Cocos	Fu ling	茯 苓
Radix Pseudostellariae Heterophyllae	Tai zi shen	太 子 參
Radix Scorphulariae Ning poensis	Xuan shen	玄 參
Radix Codonopsis Pilosulae	Dang shen	黨 參
Radix Trichosanthis Kirilowii	Tian hua fen	天 花 粉
Radix Rehmanniae	Sheng di huang	生 地 黄
Radix Rehmanniae Glutinosae Conquitae	Shu di huang	熟 地 黄
Frutus Ligustri Lucidi	Nu zhen zi	女 貞 子
Redix Glycyrrhizae Uralensis	Gan cao	甘 草
Frutus Schisandrae Chinensis	Wu wei zi	五 味 子

Tonify Qi

INGREDIENTS

Radix Astragali Membranalis	Huang qi	黄 耆
Radix Ginseng	Ji lin shen	吉 林 參
Eleutheroginseng	Wu jia shen	五 加 參
Rhizoma Atractylodis Macrocephalae	Bai zhu	白 朮
Frutus Schisandrae Chinensis	Wu wei zi	五 味 子
Redix Glycyrrhizae Uralensis	Gan cao	甘 草
Percarpium citri Reticulatae	Chen pi	陳 皮
Fructus Citri Aurantii	Zhi ke	枳 殼

Unlocking the Gate

INGREDIENTS

Saw palmetto fruit concentrate		
Radix Dioscoreae Oppositae	Shan yao	山 藥
Rhizoma Dioscoreae Hypogloaucae	Bei xie	萆 薢
Folium Pyrroisae	Shi wei	石 葦
Fructus Corni Officinalis	Shan zhu yu	山 茱 萸
Radix Achyranthis Bidentatae	Niu xi	牛 膝
Sclerotium Poriae Cocos	Fu ling	茯 苓
Rhizoma Alismatis Plantago-aquaticae	Ze xie	澤 瀉
Semen Plantaginis	Che qian zi	車 前 子
Succinum	Hu po	琥 珀
Spora Lygodii Japonici	Hai jin sha	海 金 沙
Herba Taraxaci Mongolici cum Radice	Pu gong ying	蒲 公 英
Rhizoma Smilacis	Tu fu ling	土 茯 苓
Fructus Gardiniae Jasminoidis	Shan zhi zi	山 梔 子
Cortex Phellodendri	Huang bai	黄 柏

Windbreaker

INGREDIENTS

Flos Chrysanthemi Morifolii	Huang ju hua	黃 菊 花
Herba cum Radice Asari	Xi xin	細 辛
Flos Magnoliae liliflor	Xin yi hua	辛 荑 花
Radix Puerariae	Ge gen	葛 根
Fructus Forsythiae Suspensae	Lian qiao	連 翹
Flos Lonicerae Japonicae	Jin yin hua	金 銀 花
Radix Angelicae	Bai zhi	白 芷
Herba Menthae	Bo he	薄 荷
Percarpium citri Reticulatae	Chen pi	陳 皮
Rhizoma Pinelliae Ternatae	Fa ban xia	法 半 夏
Radix Ledebouriellae Sesloidis	Fang feng	防 風
Herba seu Flos Schizonepetae Tenuifoliae	Jing jie	荆 芥
Redix Glycyrrhizae Uralensis	Gan cao	甘 草
Rhizoma Phragmitis Communis	Lu gen	蘆 根
Rhizoma Imperatae Cylincricae	Bai mao gen	白 茅 根
Radix Platycodi Grandiflori	Jie geng	桔 梗
Rhizoma et Radix Notopterygii	Qiang huo	羌 活
Folium Mori Albae	Sang ye	桑 葉
Folium Perillae Frutescentis	Zi su ye	紫 蘇 葉
Rhizoma Cimicifugae	Sheng ma	升 麻
Fructus Arctii Lappae	Niu bang zi	牛 蒡 子

Wise Woman's Well

INGREDIENTS

Gelatinum Asini	E jiao	阿 膠
Gelatinum Plastri Testudinis	Gui ban jiao	龜 板 膠
Herba Leonuri Heterophylli	Yi mu cao	益 母 草
Fluoritum	Zi shi ying	紫 石 英
Radix Anemarrhenae	Zhi mu	知 母
Os Draconis	Long gu	龍 骨
Concha Ostreae	Mu li	牡 蠣
Radix Dioscoreae Oppositae	Shan yao	山 藥

INGREDIENTS CONTINUED FROM PAGE 134

Frutus Schisandrae Chinensis	Wu wei zi	五 味 子
Caput Radicis Angelicae Sinensis	Dang gui tou	當 歸 頭
Rhizoma Atractylodis Macrocephalae	Bai zhu	白 朮
Radix Ginseng	Ji lin shen	吉 林 參
Herba Epimedii	Yin yang huo	淫 羊 藿
Semen Zizyphi Spinosae	Suan zao ren	酸 棗 仁
Caulis Polygoni Multiflori	Ye jiao teng	夜 交 藤
Semen Nelumbins	Lian zi	蓮 子
Cortex Phellodendri	Huang bai	黃 柏
Rhizoma Alismatis Plantago-aquaticae	Ze xie	澤 瀉
Rhizoma Curculiginis	Xian mao	仙 茅
Cortex Cinnamoni Cassiae	Rou gui	肉 桂

East Tao Herb Pharmacy

A.V.A.

INGREDIENTS

Herba Andrographitis Paniculatae	Chuan xin lian	穿 心 蓮
Radix Scutellariae Baicalensis	Huang qin	黃 芩
Rhizoma Coptidis	Huang lian	黃 連
Flos Lonicerae Japonicae	Jin yin hua	金 銀 花
Radix Scrophulariae Ningpoensis	Xuan shen	玄 參
Radix Isatidis seu Baphicacanthi	Ban lan gen	板 蘭 根
Rhizoma Cimicifugae	Sheng ma	升 麻
Radix Bupleuri	Chai hu	柴 胡
Fructus Forsythiae Suspensae	Lian qiao	連 翹

A.V.B.

INGREDIENTS

Radix Rehmannai	Di huang	地 黃
Radix Paeoniae Lactiflorae	Bai shao	白 芍
Cortex Moutan Radicis	Mu dan pi	牡 丹 皮
Flos Lonicerae Japonicae	Jin yin hua	金 銀 花
Rhizoma Coptidis	Huang lian	黃 連
Radix Scorphulariae Ning poensis	Xuan shen	玄 參
Fructus Forsythiae Suspensae	Lian qiao	連 翹
Radix Lithospermi seu Arnebiae	Zi cao	紫 草
Flos Carthami Tinctorii	Hong hua	紅 花
Radix Scutellariae Baicalensis	Huang qin	黃 芩

A.V.D.

INGREDIENTS

Herba Agastaches seu Pogostemi	Huo xiang	藿 香
Semen Pruni Armeniacae	Ku xing ren	苦 杏 仁
Fructus Amomi	Sha ren	砂 仁
Cortex Magnoliae Offcinalis	Hou po	厚 樸
Caulis Mutong	Mu tong	木 通
Rhizoma Acori Graminei	Shi chang pu	石 菖 蒲
Radix Scutellariae Baicalensis	Huang qin	黃 芩
Radix Bupleuri	Chai hu	柴 胡
Herba Artemisiae Yinchenhao	Yin chen	茵 陳

B-Plus (Burdock Plus)

INGREDIENTS

Ramulus Cinnamomi	Gui zhi	桂 枝
Herba Ephedrae	Ma huang	麻 黃
Fructus Xanthii Sivirici	Cang er zi	蒼 耳 子
Fructus Arctii Lappae	Niu bang zi	牛 蒡 子
Herba Menthae	Bo he	薄 荷
Radix Isatidis seu Baphicacanthi	Ban lan gen	板 蘭 根

Fructus Forsythiae Suspensae	Lian qiao	連 翹
Flos Lonicerae Japonicae	Jin yin hua	金 銀 花
Rhizoma Atractylodis Macrocephalae	Bai zhu	白 朮
Radix Bupleuri	Chai hu	柴 胡

Bi Syndrome Formula

INGREDIENTS

Rhizoma et Radix Notopterygii	Qiang huo	羌 活
Radix Angelicae Pubescentis	Du huo	獨 活
Radix Gentianae Macrophyllae	Qin jiao	秦 艽
Fructus Chaenomelis	Mu gua	木 瓜
Cortex Eucommiae Ulmoidis	Du zhong	杜 仲
Cortex Acanthopanacis Gracilistyli Radiis	Wu jia pi	五 加 皮
Radix Morindae Officinalis	Ba ji tian	巴 戟 天
Radix Aristolochiae seu Cocculi	Guang fang ji	廣 防 己
Radix Angelicae Sinensis	Dang gui	當 歸
Radix Ligustici Wallichii	Chuan xiong	川 芎
Radix Angelicae	Bai zhi	白 芷

Chahi Hu Shu Gan San Plus

INGREDIENTS

Radix Bupleuri	Chai hu	柴 胡
Radix Paeoniae Lactiflorae	Bai shao	白 芍
Fructus Citri Aurantii	Zhi ke	枳 殼
Radix Glycyrrhizae Uralensis	Gan cao	甘 草
Rhizoma Cyperi Rotudi	Xiang fu	香 附
Radix Ligustici Wallichii	Chuan xiong	川 芎
Radix Angelicae Sinensis	Dang gui	當 歸
Cortex Albizziae Julibrissin	He huan pi	合 歡 皮
Fructus Meliae Toosendan	Chuan lian zi	川 楝 子

Cleansing Formula Extract Powder

INGREDIENTS

Radix Lithospermi seu Arnebiae	Zi cao	紫草
Radix Polygoni Multiflori	Shou wu	首烏
Rhizoma Pineliae Ternatae	Ban xia	半夏
Semen Coicis	Yi yi ren	薏苡仁
Rhizoma Atractylodis Macrocephalae	Bai zhu	白朮
Sclerotium Poriae Cocos	Fu ling	茯苓
Radix Astragali	Huang qi	黃耆
Radix Rehmanniae Glutinosae	Sheng di huang	生地黃
Radix Bupleuri	Chai hu	柴胡
Radix Salviae Miltiorrhizae	Dan shen	丹參

D.U. Compound

INGREDIENTS

Radix Sanguisorbae Officinalis	Di yu	地榆
Fructus Sophorae Japonica	Huai jiao	槐角
Radix Rehmannai	Di huang	地黃
Radix Pseudoginseng	San qi	三七
Radix Scrophulariae Ningpoensis	Xuan shen	玄參
Rhizoma Cimicifugae	Sheng ma	升麻
Flos Lonicerae Japonicae	Yin hua	銀花
Fructus Forsythiae Suspensae	Lian qiao	連翹
Radix Bupleuri	Chai hu	柴胡
Radix Astragali	Huang qi	黃耆
Rhizoma Arisaematis Consanguineum	Tian nan xing	天南星
Radix Lithospermi seu Arnebiae	Zi cao	紫草

Energy A

INGREDIENTS

Radix Rehmanniae Glutinosae Conquitae	Shu di huang	熟 地 黄
Radix Astragali	Huang qi	黄 耆
Radix Angelicae Sinensis	Dang gui	當 歸
Radix Ginseng	Ren shen	人 參
Radix Paeoniae Lactiflorae	Bai shao	白 芍
Fructus Schissandra	Wu wei zi	五 味 子
Radix Salviae Miltiorrhizae	Dan shen	丹 參
Radix Glycyrrhizae Uralensis	Gan cao	甘 草
Radix Polygoni Multiflori	Shou wu	首 烏
Cortex Acanthopanacis Gracilistyli Radiis	Wu jia pi	五 加 皮

Energy C

INGREDIENTS

Tuber Ophiopogonis Japonici	Mai men dong	麥 門 冬
Radix Scrophulariae Ningpoensis	Xuan shen	玄 參
Radix Panacis Quinquefolii	Xi yang shen	西 洋 參
Radix Adenophorae Tetraphylla	Nan sha shen	南 沙 參
Radix Trichosanthis Kirilowii	Tian hua fen	天 花 粉
Frutus Schisandrae Chinensis	Wu wei zi	五 味 子
Radix Puerariae	Ge gen	葛 根
Radix Anemarrhenae	Zhi mu	知 母

Energy D

INGREDIENTS

Cortex Eucommiae Ulmoidis	Du zhong	杜 仲
Radix Morindae Officinalis	Ba ji tian	巴 戟 天
Fructus Rosae	Jin ying zi	金 櫻 子
Fructus Rubi Chingii	Fu pen zi	覆 盆 子
Fructus Alpiniae Oxyphyllae	Yi zhi ren	益 智 仁
Frutus Schisandrae Chinensis	Wu wei zi	五 味 子
Cortex Cinnamomi Cassiae	Rou gui	肉 桂
Radix Ginseng	Ren shen	人 參

Energy E

INGREDIENTS

Radix Bupleuri	Chai hu	柴 胡
Radix Ginseng	Ren shen	人 參
Radix Codonopsis Pilosulae	Dang shen	黨 參
Radix Paeoniae Lactiflorae	Bai shao	白 芍
Sclerotium Poriae Cocos	Fu ling	茯 苓
Fructus Citri Aurantii	Zhi ke	枳 殼
Rhizoma Atractylodis	Bai zhu	白 朮
Rhizoma Cyperus Rotundi	Xiang fu	香 附
Radix Angelicae Sinensis	Dang gui	當 歸
Cortex Magnoliae Officinalis	Hou po	厚 樸

Energy K

INGREDIENTS

Radix Codonopsitis Pilosulae	Dang shen	黨 參
Radix Ginseng	Ren shen	人 參
Rhizoma Atractylodis Macrocephalae	Bai zhu	白 朮
Radix Puerariae	Ge gen	葛 根
Radix Bupleuri	Chai hu	柴 胡
Rhizoma Cimicifugae	Sheng ma	升 麻
Frutus Schisandrae Chinensis	Wu wei zi	五 味 子
Fructus Evodiae	Wu zhu yu	吳 茱 萸
Radix Aucklandiae Lappae	Mu xiang	木 香
Radix Astragali	Huang qi	黃 耆
Pericarpium Citri Reticulatae	Chen pi	陳 皮
Radix Glycyrrhizae Uralensis	Gan cao	甘 草

Energy L

INGREDIENTS

Radix Ginseng	Ren shen	人參
Radix Angelicae Sinensis	Dang gui	當歸
Fructus Lycii Chinensis	Gou qi zi	枸杞子
Radix Achyranthis Bidentatae	Niu xi	牛膝
Radix Polygoni Multiflori	Shou wu	首烏
Fructus Corni Officinalis	Shan zhu yu	山茱萸
Cortex Eucommiae Ulmoidis	Du zhong	杜仲
Semen Astraguli Complanati	Sha yuan ji zi	沙苑蒺子
Radix Rehmanniae Glutinosae Conquitae	Shu di huang	熟地黃
Semen Cuscutae	Tu si zi	兎絲子
Herba Cistanches	Rou cong rong	肉蓯蓉
Plastrum Testudinis	Gui ban	龜板

Energy S

INGREDIENTS

Radix Rehmanniae Glutinosae	Sheng di huang	生地黃
Excrementum Trogopteri seu Pteromi	Wu ling zhi	五靈脂
Radix Angelicae Sinensis	Dang gui	當歸
Eleutheroginseng	Wu jia shen	五加參
Radix Ginseng	Ren shen	人參
Semen Ziziphi	Suan zao ren	酸棗仁
Arillus Euphoriae Longanae	Long yan rou	龍眼肉
Radix Salviae Miltiorrhizae	Dan shen	丹參

Er Xian Tang Plus

INGREDIENTS

Herba Epimedii	Yin yang huo	淫羊藿
Radix Morindae Officinalis	Ba ji tian	巴戟天
Cortex Eucommiae Ulmoidis	Du zhong	杜仲
Radix Achyranthis Bidentatae	Niu xi	牛膝
Radix Anemarrhenae	Zhi mu	知母

INGREDIENTS CONTINUED FROM PAGE 141

Radix Ginseng	Ren shen	人參
Radix Astragali	Huang qi	黃耆
Radix Angelicae Sinensis	Dang gui	當歸
Fructus Corni Officinalis	Shan zhu yu	山茱萸

Flavor 21–Capsules

INGREDIENTS

Radix Notoginseng	San qi	三七
Radix Ginseng	Ren shen	人參
Radix Angelicae Sinensis	Dang gui	當歸
Radix Polygoni Multiflori	Shou wu	首烏
Rhizoma Coptidis	Huang lian	黃連
Cortex Moutan Radicis	Mu dan pi	牡丹皮
Radix Scutellariae Baicalensis	Huang qin	黃芩
Rhizoma Curcumae zedoariae	E zhu	莪朮
Cortex Phellodendri	Huang bai	黃柏
Radix Gentianae Macrophyllae	Qin jiao	秦艽
Myrrha	Mo yao	沒藥
Fructus Gardeniae Jasminoidis	Shan zhi zi	山梔子
Rhizoma Sparganii	San leng	三稜
Radix Glycyrrhizae Uralensis	Gan cao	甘草
Radix Salviae Miltiorrhizae	Dan shen	丹參
Radix et Rhizoma Rhei	Da huang	大黃
Fructus Zizyphi Jujubae	Da zao	大棗
Herba Ephedrae	Ma huang	麻黃
Rhizoma Zingiberis Officialis Recens	Sheng jiang	生姜
Indigo Naturalis		

G. Plus (Gastropodia Plus) Tablets

INGREDIENTS

Rhizoma Gastrodiae Elatae	Tian ma	天 麻
Flos Chrysanthemi Morifolii	Huang ju hua	黄 菊 花
Folium Mori Albae	Sang ye	桑 葉
Os Draconis	Long gu	龍 骨
Concha Ostreae	Mu li	牡 蠣
Haematitum	Dai zhe shi	代 赭 石
Spica Prunellae Vulgaris	Xia ku cao	夏 枯 草

Gentiana Compound

INGREDIENTS

Radix Gentianae Scabrae	Long dan cao	龍 膽 草
Radix Scutellariae Baicalensis	Huang qin	黄 芩
Rhizoma Coptidis	Huang lian	黄 連
Caulis Akebiae	Mu tong	木 通
Sclerotium Poriae Cocos	Fu ling	茯 苓
Radix Sophorae Flavescentis	Ku shen	苦 參
Radix Cyathulae	Chuan niu xi	川 牛 膝
Cortex Phellodendri	Huang bai	黄 柏
Rhizoma Alismatis Plantago-aquaticae	Ze xie	澤 瀉

Ginkgo Compound

INGREDIENTS

Folium Ginkgo Bilobae	Bai guo ye	白 果 葉
Radix Puerariae	Ge gen	葛 根
Radix Salviae Miltiorrhizae	Dan shen	丹 參
Radix Ginseng	Ren shen	人 參
Cortex Acanthopanacis Gracilistyli Radiis	Wu jia pi	五 加 皮
Frutus Schisandrae Chinensis	Wu wei zi	五 味 子
Ganodermae Lucidum	Ling zhi	靈 芝

Golden Balm Spray or Paste

INGREDIENTS

Rhizoma Coptidis	Huang lian	黄 連
Radix Scutellariae Baicalensis	Huang qin	黄 芩
Radix Sophorae Flavescentis	Ku shen	苦 參
Borneol	Bing pian	冰 片
Calculus Bovis	Niu huang	牛 黄
Scretio Bufonis	Chan su	蟾 酥
Radix Pseudoginseng	San qi	三 七
Borax		
Indigo pulverata levis		

Golden Rose

INGREDIENTS

Radix Sophorae Flavescentis	Ku shen	苦 參
Radix Gentianae Macrophyllae	Qin jiao	秦 艽
Cortex Phellodendri	Huang bai	黄 柏
Rhizoma Atractyloidis	Cang zhu	蒼 朮
Sclerotium Poriae Cocos	Fu ling	茯 苓
Herba Agastaches seu Pogostemi	Huo xiang	藿 香
Radix et Caulis Jixueteng	Ji xue teng	雞 血 藤

Green Xiao Yao San

INGREDIENTS

Radix Bupleuri	Chai hu	柴 胡
Radix Paeoniae Lactiflorae	Bai shao	白 芍
Fructus Immaturus Citri Aurantii	Zhi shi	枳 實
Radix Glycyrrhizae Uralensis	Gan cao	甘 草
Rhizoma Cyperi Rotudi	Xiang fu	香 附
Tuber Curcumae	Yu jin	郁 金
Radix Aucklandiae Lappae	Mu xiang	木 香
Herba Aloes	Lu hui	蘆 薈
Radix Gentianae Macrophyllae	Qin jiao	秦 艽

Radix et Rhizoma Rhei	Da huang	大 黃
Radix Scutellariae Baicalensis	Huang qin	黃 芩
Sulfuricum Natrium	Mang xiao	芒 硝

Heaven Age Tea

INGREDIETNTS

Radix Polygoni Multiflori	Shou wu	首 烏
Radix Ginseng	Ren shen	人 參
Radix Angelicae Sinensis	Dang gui	當 歸
Radix Rehmanniae	Di huang	地 黃
Radix Salviae Miltiorrhizae	Dan shen	丹 參
Folium Ginkgo Bilobae	Bai guo ye	白 果 葉
Fructus Lycii Chinensis	Gou qi zi	枸 杞 子
Radix Puerariae	Ge gen	葛 根
Frutus Schisandrae Chinensis	Wu wei zi	五 味 子
Excrementum Trogopteri seu Pteromi	Wu ling zhi	五 靈 脂
Cortex Acanthopanacis Gracilistyli Radiis	Wu jia pi	五 加 皮
Radix Pseudoginseng	San qi	三 七
Rhizoma Dioscoreae Hypogloaucae	Bei xie	萆 薢
Frutus Mori Albae	Sang shen	桑 椹

Isatis Compound

INGREDIENTS

Radix Isatidis seu Baphicacanthi	Ban lan gen	板 蘭 根
Radix Sophorae Flavescentis	Ku shen	苦 參
Flos Lonicerae Japonicae	Yin hua	銀 花
Radix Scutellariae Baicalensis	Huang qin	黃 芩
Herba Andrographitis Paniculatae	Chuan xin lian	穿 心 蓮
Fructus Forsythiae Suspensae	Lian qiao	連 翹
Radix Bupleuri	Chai hu	柴 胡
Rhizoma Pinelliae Ternatae	Fa ban xia	法 半 夏
Radix Glycyrrhizae Uralensis	Zhi gan cao	炙 甘 草
Indigo		

Jade Screen

INGREDIENTS

Radix Astragali	Huang qi	黄 耆
Radix Ginseng	Ren shen	人 參
Radix Paeoniae	Shao yao	芍 藥
Frutus Schisandrae Chinensis	Wu wei zi	五 味 子
Rhizoma Atractylodis Macrocephalae	Bai zhu	白 朮
Radix Ledebouriellae Sesloidis	Fang feng	防 風
Ramulus Cinnamomi	Gui zhi	桂 枝
Radix Glycyrrhizae Uralensis	Gan cao	甘 草
Echinacea purpura		

Jade Shining

INGREDIENTS

Cortex Acanthopanacis Gracilistyli Radiis	Wu jia pi	五 加 皮
Fructus Lycii Chinensis	Gou qi zi	枸 杞 子
Semen Cuscutae	Tu si zi	兔 絲 子
Radix Angelicae Sinensis	Dang gui	當 歸
Radix Astragali	Huang qi	黄 耆
Radix Lithospermi seu Arnebiae	Zi cao	紫 草
Radix Polygoni Multiflori	Shou wu	首 烏
Radix Rehmanniae Glutinosae Conquitae	Shu di huang	熟 地 黄
Rhizoma Dioscoreae Hypogloaucae	Bei xie	萆 薢
Rhizoma Polygoni Cuspidati	Hu zhang	虎 杖

Light Clearing

INGREDIENTS

Flos Lonicerae Japonicae	Jin yin hua	金 銀 花
Radix Ligustici Wallichii	Chuan xiong	川 芎
Herba seu Flos Schizonepetae Tenuifoliae	Jing jie	荆 芥
Fructus Viticis	Man jing zi	蔓 荆 子
Herba Menthae	Bo he	薄 荷

INGREDIENTS CONTINUED FROM PAGE 146

Radix Ledebouriellae Sesloidis	Fang feng	防 風
Fructus Tribuli Terrestris	Bai ji li	白 蒺 藜
Radix Angelicae Sinensis	Dang gui	當 歸
Flos Chrysanthemi Morifolii	Ju hua	菊 花
Fructus Xanthii Sivirici	Cang er zi	蒼 耳 子
Fructus Forsythiae Suspensae	Lian qiao	連 翹

Ling Syndrome Formula

INGREDIENTS

Rhizoma Dioscoreae Hypogloaucae	Bei xie	萆 薢
Radix Linderae Strychnifoliae	Wu yao	烏 藥
Caulis Mutong	Mu tong	木 通
Sclerotium Polypori Umbellati	Zhu ling	豬 苓
Radix Rehmannai	Di huang	地 黃
Fructus Alpiniae Oxyphyllae	Yi zhi ren	益 智 仁
Herba Lysimachiae	Jin qian cao	金 錢 草
Radix Sophorae Flavescentis	Ku shen	苦 參
Radix Salviae Miltiorrhizae	Dan shen	丹 參

Lou-Bu-Ma Compound

INGREDIENTS

Herba seu Folium Apocym Vendti	Luo bu ma	羅 布 麻
Cortex Eucommiae Ulmoidis	Du zhong	杜 仲
Ramulus Uncariae cum Uncis	Gou teng	鉤 藤
Rhizoma Gastrodiae Elatae	Tian ma	天 麻
Radix Ligustici Wallichii	Chuan xiong	川 芎
Radix Salviae Miltiorrhizae	Dan shen	丹 參
Radix Puerariae	Ge gen	葛 根
Semen Ginkgo	Bai guo	白 果
Radix Paeoniae Lactiflorae	Bai shao	白 芍
Radix Cyathulae	Chuan niu xi	川 牛 膝

Lotus Balm

INGREDIENTS

Fructus Cnidii	She chuang zi	蛇床子
Radix Sophorae	Ku shen	苦參
Flos Daphnes	Yuan hua	芫花
Cortex Phellodendri	Huang bai	黃柏
Fructus Gleditsiae	Zhu ya zao	豬牙皂

Morning Glory

INGREDIENTS

Cortex Magnoliae Offcinalis	Hou po	厚樸
Fructus Citri Aurantii	Zhi ke	枳殼
Fructus Crataegi	Shan zha	山楂
Fructus Forsythiae Suspensae	Lian qiao	連翹
Pericarpium Citri Reticulatae	Chen pi	陳皮
Radix Picrorrhizae	Hu huang lian	胡黃連
Rhizoma Pinelliae Ternatae	Fa ban xia	法半夏
Semen Arecae Catechu	Bing lang	檳榔
Semen Pharbitidis	Qian niu zi	牽牛子
Digestive Enzyme		

Mountain Sophora

INGREDIENTS

Moutain Sophora		
Indigo		
Radix Platycodi Grandiflora	Jie geng	桔梗
Rhizoma Belamcamdae Chinensis	She gan	射干
Radix Glycyrrhizae Uralensis	Gan cao	甘草
Radix Scutellariae Baicalensis	Huang qin	黃芩
Borneol	Bing pian	冰片
Herba Menthae	Bo he	薄荷

Pang Da Hai Compound-Extract Powder

INGREDIENTS

Semen Sterculiae Scaphigerae	Pang da hai	胖大海
Fructus Terminaliae Chebulae	He zi	訶子
Radix Sophorae Flavescentis	Ku shen	苦參
Bulbus Fritillariae Thunbergii	Zhe bei mu	浙貝母
Radix Trichosanthis Kirilowii	Tian hua fen	天花粉
Rhizoma Belamcamdae Chinensis	She gan	射干
Semen Pruni Armeniacae	Ku xing ren	苦杏仁
Rhizoma Pinelliae Ternatae	Fa ban xia	法半夏
Radix Glycyrrhizae Uralensis	Gan cao	甘草
Radix Platycodi Grandiflora	Jie geng	桔梗
Radix Scrophulariae Ningpoensis	Xuan shen	玄參

PHL-I

INGREDIENTS

Pericarpium Citri Reticulatae	Chen pi	陳皮
Rhizoma Pinelliae Ternatae	Fa ban xia	法半夏
Sclerotium Poriae Cocos	Fu ling	茯苓
Radix Glycyrrhizae Uralensis	Gan cao	甘草
Rhizoma Arisaematis Consanguineum	Tian nan xing	天南星
Fructus Immaturus Citri Aurantii	Zhi shi	枳實
Cortex Magnoliae Offcinalis	Hou po	厚樸
Herba cum Raice Asari	Xi xin	細辛
Flos Tussilaginis Farfarae	Kuan dong hua	款冬花
Radix Platycodi Grandiflora	Jie geng	桔梗

Ping Wei San Plus

INGREDIENTS

Cortex Magnoliae Offcinalis	Hou po	厚樸
Rhizoma Atractylodis Macrocephalae	Bai zhu	白朮
Pericarpium Citri Reticulatae	Chen pi	陳皮
Radix Glycyrrhizae Uralensis	Gan cao	甘草

INGREDIENTS CONTINUED FROM PAGE 149

Herba Agastaches seu Pogostemi	Huo xiang	藿 香
Folium Perillae Frutescentis	Su ye	蘇 葉
Radix Paeoniae Lactiflorae	Bai shao	白 芍
Rhizoma Pinelliae Ternatae	Fa ban xia	法 半 夏
Radix Saussureae seu Vladimiriae	Mu xiang	木 香
Rhizoma Cyperi Rotudi	Xiang fu	香 附
Fructus Evodiae	Wu zhu yu	吳 茱 萸
Rhizoma Zingiberis Officialis Recens	Sheng jiang	生 姜

Q.B.A.

INGREDIENTS

Radix Paeoniae Lactiflorae	Bai shao	白 芍
Flos Carthami Tinctorii	Hong hua	紅 花
Fructus Citri Aurantii	Zhi ke	枳 殼
Radix Salviae Miltiorrhizae	Dan shen	丹 參
Cortex Moutan Radicis	Mu dan pi	牡 丹 皮
Radix Platycodi Grandiflora	Jie geng	桔 梗
Radix Ligustici Wallichii	Chuan xiong	川 芎
Fructus Meliae Toosendan	Chuan lian zi	川 楝 子

Q.B.H.

INGREDIENTS

Radix Trichosanthis	Gua lou gen	瓜 蔞 根
Flos Lonicerae Japonicae	Yin hua	銀 花
Radix Angelicae Dahuricae	Bai zhi	白 芷
Radix Angelicae Sinensis	Dang gui	當 歸
Radix Paeoniae Lactiflorae	Bai shao	白 芍
Spina Gleditsiae Sinensis	Zao jiao ci	皂 角 刺
Spica Prunellae Vulgaris	Xia ku cao	夏 枯 草
Radix Bupleuri	Chai hu	柴 胡
Radix Scrophulariae Ningpoensis	Xuan shen	玄 參

Q.B.R.

INGREDIENTS

Cortex Moutan Radicis	Mu dan pi	牡丹皮
Radix Paeoniae Lactiflorae	Bai shao	白芍
Radix Rehmannai	Di huang	地黄
Radix Scrophulariae Ningpoensis	Xuan shen	玄參
Radix Angelicae Sinensis	Dang gui	當歸
Flos Carthami Tinctorii	Hong hua	紅花
Radix Scutellariae Baicalensis	Huang qin	黄芩
Radix Gentianae Macrophyllae	Qin jiao	秦艽
Radix Sanguisorbae Officinalis	Di yu	地榆
Radix Lithospermi seu Arnebiae	Zi cao	紫草

Q.B.S.

INGREDIENTS

Rhizoma Coptidis	Huang lian	黄連
Radix Scutellariae Baicalensis	Huang qin	黄芩
Cortex Phellodendri	Huang bai	黄柏
Fructus Gardeniae Jasminoidis	Shan zhi zi	山梔子
Radix Gentianae Macrophyllae	Qin jiao	秦艽
Flos Lonicerae Japonicae	Yin hua	銀花
Radix Bupleuri	Chai hu	柴胡
Radix Rehmannai	Di huang	地黄
Indigo Pulverata levis		

Q.B.Y.

INGREDIENTS

Radix Paeoniae Lactiflorae	Bai shao	白芍
Radix Salviae Miltiorrhizae	Dan shen	丹參
Radix Achyranthis Bidentatae	Niu xi	牛膝
Radix Puerariae	Ge gen	葛根
Radix Scrophulariae Ningpoensis	Xuan shen	玄參
Haematitum	Dai zhe shi	代赭石

INGREDIENTS CONTINUED FROM PAGE 151

Plastrum Testudinis	Gui ban	龜 板
Os Draconis	Long gu	龍 骨
Radix Scutellariae Baicalensis	Huang qin	黃 芩
Radix Rehmannai	Di huang	地 黃

R-Plus (Peach Seed Plus)

INGREDIENTS

Semen Persicae	Tao ren	桃 仁
Semen Pruni Armeniacae	Ku xing ren	苦 杏 仁
Semen Pruni	Yu li ren	郁 李 仁
Flos Carthami Tinctorii	Hong hua	紅 花
Radix Codonopsis Pilosulae	Dang shen	黨 參
Radix Paeoniae Lactiflorae	Bai shao	白 芍
Herba Aloes	Lu hui	蘆 薈
Radix Ginseng	Ren shen	人 參
Radix Astragali	Huang qi	黃 耆
Radix Bupleuri	Chai hu	柴 胡
Cortex Magnoliae Offcinalis	Hou po	厚 樸
Radix Ledebouriellae Sesloidis	Fang feng	防 風

R.D.A

INGREDIENTS

Rhizoma et Radix Notopterygii	Qiang huo	羌 活
Radix Angelicae	Bai zhi	白 芷
Radix Ledebouriellae Sesloidis	Fang feng	防 風
Herba cum Raice Asari	Xi xin	細 辛
Rhizoma Atractylodis Macrocephalae	Bai zhu	白 朮
Radix Angelicae Sinensis	Dang gui	當 歸
Radix Ligustici Wallichii	Chuan xiong	川 芎
Ramulus Cinnamomi	Gui zhi	桂 枝
Radix Clematidis	Wei ling xian	威 靈 仙

R.D.Y.

INGREDIENTS

Radix Gentianae Scabrae	Long dan cao	龍 膽 草
Radix Bupleuri	Chai hu	柴 胡
Radix Scutellariae Baicalensis	Huang qin	黄 芩
Radix Rehmannai	Di huang	地 黄
Caulis Mutong	Mu tong	木 通
Rhizoma Alismatis Plantago-aquaticae	Ze xie	澤 瀉
Fructus Gardeniae Jasminoidis	Shan zhi zi	山 梔 子
Radix Achyranthis Bidentatae	Niu xi	牛 膝
Radix Sophorae Flavescentis	Ku shen	苦 參
Spica Prunellae Vulgaris	Xia ku cao	夏 枯 草
Cortex Phellodendri	Huang bai	黄 柏

Shao Yang Formula

INGREDIENTS

Radix Bupleuri	Chai hu	柴 胡
Rhizoma Pinelliae Ternatae	Fa ban xia	法 半 夏
Radix Ginseng	Ren shen	人 參
Radix Scutellariae Baicalensis	Huang qin	黄 芩
Fructus Evodiae	Wu zhu yu	吳 茱 萸
Radix Pseudoginseng	San qi	三 七
Pericarpium Citri Reticulatae	Chen pi	陳 皮
Fructus Immaturus Citri Aurantii	Zhi shi	枳 實
Caulis Bambusae in Taeniis	Zhu ru	竹 茹
Rhizoma Coptidis	Huang lian	黄 連

Sheng Mai San Plus

INGREDIENTS

Radix Ginseng	Ren shen	人 參
Tuber Ophiopogonis Japonici	Mai men dong	麥 門 冬
Frutus Schisandrae Chinensis	Wu wei zi	五 味 子
Radix Astragali	Huang qi	黃 耆
Rhizoma Atractylodis Macrocephalae	Bai zhu	白 朮
Radix Paeoniae Lactiflorae	Bai shao	白 芍

Shu Xie Tea

INGREDIENTS

Radix Bupleuri	Chai hu	柴 胡
Rhizoma Cyperi Rotudi	Xiang fu	香 附
Fructus Meliae Toosendan	Chuan lian zi	川 楝 子
Radix Angelicae Sinensis	Dang gui	當 歸
Radix Paeoniae Lactiflorae	Bai shao	白 芍
Pericarpium Citri Reticulatae	Chen pi	陳 皮
Radix Salviae Miltiorrhizae	Dan shen	丹 參
Cortex Albizziae Julibrissin	He huan pi	合 歡 皮
Radix Ligustici Wallichii	Chuan xiong	川 芎
Excrementum Trogopteri seu Pteromi	Wu ling zhi	五 靈 脂

Smilax

INGREDIENTS

Rhizoma Smilacis	Tu fu ling	土 茯 苓
Radix Glycyrrhizae Uralensis	Gan cao	甘 草
Radix Clematidis	Wei ling xian	威 靈 仙
Radix Pseudoginseng	San qi	三 七
Flos Carthami Tinctorii	Hong hua	紅 花
Radix Angelicae Sinensis	Dang gui	當 歸
Fructus Chaenomelis	Mu gua	木 瓜
Radix Sarcandrae	Zhong jie feng	腫 節 風

Tian Kui T-F

INGREDIENTS

Cortex Eucommiae Ulmoidis	Du zhong	杜仲
Fructus Corni Officinalis	Shan zhu yu	山茱萸
Frutus Schisandrae Chinensis	Wu wei zi	五味子
Herba Leonuri Heterophylli	Yi mu cao	益母草
Radix Angelicae Sinensis	Dang gui	當歸
Radix Rehmanniae Glutinosae Conquitae	Shu di huang	熟地黃
Rhizoma Cyperi Rotudi	Xiang fu	香附
Wild yam		

Tian Kui T-M

INGREDIENTS

Radix Ginseng	Ren shen	人參
Cornu Cervi Parvum	Lu rong	鹿茸
Herba Cistanches	Rou cong rong	肉蓯蓉
Semen Cuscutae	Tu si zi	菟絲子
Fructus Cnidii	She chuang zi	蛇床子
Fructus Corni Officinalis	Shan zhu yu	山茱萸
Fructus Viticis	Man jing zi	蔓荊子
Semen Astragali Complanati	Sha yuan zi	沙苑子
Herba Cynomorii Songarici	Suo yang	鎖陽
Radix Morindae Officinalis	Ba ji tian	巴戟天

White Flower

INGREIENTS

Herba Hendyotidis		
Pseudobulbus		
Rhizoma Curcumae zedoariae	E zhu	莪朮
Cortex Moutan Radicis	Mu dan pi	牡丹皮
Ramulus Cinnamomi	Gui zhi	桂枝
Radix Sophorae Flavescentis	Ku shen	苦參
Rhizoma Arisaematis Consanguineum	Tian nan xing	天南星
Radix Astragali	Huang qi	黃耆

Wolfberry Compound-Extract Powder

INGREDIENTS

Flos Chrysanthemi Morifolii	Ju hua	菊 花
Fructus Tribuli Terrestris	Bai ji li	白 蒺 藜
Herba Dendrobii	Shi hu	石 斛
Radix Angelicae Sinensis	Dang gui	當 歸
Radix Gentianae Macrophyllae	Qin jiao	秦 艽
Radix Paeoniae Lactiflorae	Bai shao	白 芍
Radix Polygoni Multiflori	Shou wu	首 烏
Radix Rehmanniae Glutinosae Conquitae	Shu di huang	熟 地 黃
Radix Salviae Miltiorrhizae	Dan shen	丹 參
Semen Cassiae Torae	Jue ming zi	決 明 子
Fructus Lycii Chinensis	Gou qi zi	枸 杞 子
Radix Buffleiae		

Women's Relaxing

INGREDIENTS

Radix Bupleuri	Chai hu	柴 胡
Radix Angelicae Sinensis	Dang gui	當 歸
Herba Leonuri Heterophylli	Yi mu cao	益 母 草
Radix Paeoniae Lactiflorae	Bai shao	白 芍
Cortex Magnoliae Offcinalis	Hou po	厚 樸
Sclerotium Poriae Cocos	Fu ling	茯 苓
Flos Chrysanthemi Morifolii	Ju hua	菊 花
Radix Rehmannai	Di huang	地 黃
Rhizoma et Radix Ligustici Sinensis	Chuan xiong	川 芎
Rhizoma Atractylodis Macrocephalae	Bai zhu	白 朮

Wu Mei Wan Plus

INGREDIENTS

Frutus Schisandrae Chinensis	Wu wei zi	五味子
Herba cum Raice Asari	Xi xin	細辛
Cortex Cinnamomi Cassiae	Rou gui	肉桂
Radix Ginseng	Ren shen	人參
Radix Aconiti Carmichaelai Praeparata	Fu zi	附子
Pericarpium Zanthoxyli Bungeani	Hua jiao	花椒
Rhizoma Coptidis	Huang lian	黄連
Rhizoma Zingiberis Officialis Recens	Sheng jiang	生姜
Cortex Phellodendri	Huang bai	黄柏
Fructus Evodiae	Wu zhu yu	吳茱萸
Fructus Psorateae	Wu Mei	烏梅

X-Plus (Xanthium Plus)

INGREDIENTS

Fructus Xanthii Sivirici	Cang er zi	蒼耳子
Herba Agastaches seu Pogostemi	Huo xiang	藿香
Radix Bupleuri	Chai hu	柴胡
Herba cum Raice Asari	Xi xin	細辛
Radix Platycodi Grandiflora	Jie geng	桔梗
Radix Scutellariae Baicalensis	Huang qin	黄芩
Radix Angelicae Sinensis	Dang gui	當歸
Rhizoma Pinelliae Ternatae	Fa ban xia	法半夏
Flos Chrysanthemi Morifolii	Ju hua	菊花
Centipeda Minima	E bu shi cao	鵝不食草
Herba Menthae	Bo he	薄荷

Yellow Xiao Yao San

INGREDIENTS

Radix Bupleuri	Chai hu	柴胡
Radix Paeoniae Lactiflorae	Bai shao	白芍
Pericarpium Citri Reticulatae	Chen pi	陳皮
Radix Glycyrrhizae Uralensis	Gan cao	甘草
Rhizoma Cyperi Rotudi	Xiang fu	香附
Radix Ligustici Wallichii	Chuan xiong	川芎
Cortex Magnoliae Offcinalis	Hou po	厚樸
Rhizoma Atractylodis Macrocephalae	Bai zhu	白朮
Rhizoma Pinelliae Ternatae	Fa ban xia	法半夏
Pericarpium Citri Reticulatae	Chen pi	陳皮
Fructus seu Semen Amomi	Sha ren	砂仁
Fructus Evodiae	Wu zhu yu	吳茱萸
Rhizoma Coptidis	Huang lian	黃連
Fructus Gardeniae Jasminoidis	Shan zhi zi	山梔子

Zi Cao Compound

INGREDIENTS

Radix Lithospermi seu Arnebiae	Zi cao	紫草
Radixx Ledebouriellae Divaricatae	Fang feng	防風
Herba seu Flos Schizonepetae Tenuifoliae	Jing jie	荆芥
Fructus Forsythiae Suspensae	Lian qiao	連翹
Radix Bupleuri	Chai hu	柴胡
Radix Scrophulariae Ningpoensis	Xuan shen	玄參
Rhizoma Cimicifugae	Sheng ma	升麻
Flos Carthami Tinctorii	Hong hua	紅花
Cortex Dictamni Radicis	Bai xian pi	白蘚皮
Radix Peaoniae Rubra	Chi shao	赤芍
Radix Rehmanniae	Di huang	地黄
Radix Sairiae		

GOLDEN FLOWER CHINESE HERBS

Astralagus Formula

INGREDIENTS		
Saccharum Granorrum	Yi tang	飴糖
Ramulus Cinnamomi	Gui zhi	桂枝
Radix Paeoniae	Bai shao	白芍
Rhizoma Zingiberis Officinalis	Sheng jiang	生姜
Fructus Ziziphi Jujubae	Da zao	大棗
Honey-toasted Radix Glycyrrhizae	Zhi gan cao	炙甘草
Rhizoma Atractylodis Macrocephalae	Bai zhu	白朮
Radix Astragali	Huang qi	黄耆

Bupleurum and Tang Kuei Formula

INGREDIENTS		
Radix Bupleuri	Chai hu	柴胡
Radix Angelicae Sinensis	Dang gui	當歸
Radix Paeoniae Lactiflorae	Bai shao	白芍
Rhizoma Atractylodis Macrocephalae	Bai zhu	白朮
Poria	Fu ling	茯苓
Toasted Radix Glycyrrhizae Uralensis	Zhi gan cao	炙甘草
Rhizoma Zigiberis Officinalis	Gan jiang	乾姜
Herba Menthae	Bo he	薄荷

Bupleurum E Formula

INGREDIENTS		
Radix Bupleurum	Chai hu	柴胡
Radix Codonopsis Pilosulae	Dang shen	黨參
Rhizoma Pinelliae Ternatae	Ban xia	半夏
Radix Scutellariae Baicalensis	Huang qin	黄芩
Rhizoma Zingiberis Officinalis	Sheng jiang	生姜
Ramulus Cinnamomi Cassiae	Gui zhi	桂枝

INGREDIENTS CONTINUED FROM PAGE 159

Sclerotium Poriae Cocos Pararadicis	Fu shen	茯 神
Os Draconis	Long gu	龍 骨
Concha Ostreae	Mu li	牡 蠣
Rhizoma Rhei	Da huang	大 黃
Fructus Ziziphi Jujubae	Da zao	大 棗
Rhizoma Acori Graminei	Shi chang pu	石 菖 蒲

Chase Wind, Penetrate Bone Formula

INGREDIENTS

Mel	Feng mi	蜂 蜜
Ramulus mLoranthi seu Visci	Sang ji sheng	桑 寄 生
Rhizoma Cyperi Rou\tundi	Xiang fu	香 附
Rhizoma et Radix Notopterygii	Qiang huo	羌 活
Rhizoma et Radix Ligusti Sinensis	Gao ben	藁 本
Cortex Eucommiae Ulmoidis	Du zhong	杜 仲
Radix Achyranthis Bidentatae	Niu xi	牛 膝
Herba Asari cum Radice	Xi xin	細 辛
Radix Paeoniae Lactiflorae	Bai shao	白 芍
Radix Angelicae	Bai zhi	白 芷
Radix Dipsaci	Xu duan	續 斷
Radix Glycyrrhizae Uralensis	Gan cao	甘 草
Radix Pseudoginseng	San qi	三 七
Poria	Fu ling	茯 苓
Myrrha	Mo yao	沒 藥
Radix Duhuo	Du huo	獨 活
Cortex Cinnamomi Cassiae	Rou gui	肉 桂
Rhizoma Gastrodiae Elatae	Tian ma	天 麻
Rhizoma Nardostachytis Chinensis	Gan Song xiang	甘 松 香
Gummi Olibanum	Ru xiang	乳 香
Radix Gentianae Macrophyllae	Qin jiao	秦 艽
Radix Ledebouriellae Sesloidis	Fang feng	防 風

Cinnmon and Poria Formula

INGREDIENTS

Radix Paeoniae Rubra	Chi shao	赤 芍
Ramulus Cinnamomi Cassiae	Gui zhi	桂 枝
Poria	Fu ling	茯 苓
Cortex Moutan Radicis	Mu dan pi	牡 丹 皮
Semen Persicae	Tao ren	桃 仁
Radix Paeoniae	Bai shao	白 芍
Radix Salviae Miltiorrhizae	Dan shen	丹 參
Rhizoma Rhei	Da huang	大 黄
Rhizoma Sparganii	San leng	三 稜

Coptos Relieve Toxicity Formula

INGREDIENTS

Fructus Gardenia Jasminoidis	Zhi zi	梔 子
Rhizoma Coptidis	Huang lian	黄 連
Herba Lophatheri Gracllis	Dan zhu ye	淡 竹 葉
Radix Scutellariae Baicalensis	Huang qin	黄 芩
Cortex Phellodendri	Huang bai	黄 柏
Rhizoma Rhei	Da huang	大 黄

Corydalis Formula

INGREDIENTS

Extract of Rhizoma Corydalis	Yan hu suo	延 胡 索
Radix Paeoniae Lactiflorae	Bai shao	白 芍
Radix Glycyrrhizae Uralensis	Gan cao	甘 草

Du Huo and Loranthus Formula

INGREDIENTS

Ramulus Sangjisheng	Sang ji sheng	桑 寄 生
Radix Angelicae Pubescentis	Du huo	獨 活
Flos Carthami Tinctorii	Hong hua	紅 花
Herba cum Radice Asari	Xi xin	細 辛
Radix Ledebouriellae Divaricatae	Fang feng	防 風
Radix Gentianae Qinjiao	Qin jiao	秦 艽
Cortex Eucommiae Ulmoidis	Du zhong	杜 仲
Radix Achyranthis Bidentatae	Niu xi	牛 膝
Cortex Cinnamomi Cassiae	Rou gui	肉 桂
Radix Angelicae Sinensis	Dang gui	當 歸
Radix Paeoniae Lactiflorae	Bai shao	白 芍
Radix Ligustici Chuanxiong	Chuan xiong	川 芎
Radix Rehmanniae Glutinosae Conquitae	Shu di huang	熟 地 黄
Radix Ginseng	Ren shen	人 參
Poria	Fu ling	茯 苓
Honey-fried Radix Glycyrrhizae Uralensis	Zhi gan cao	炙 甘 草

Ease Digestion Formula

INGREDIENTS

Poria	Fu ling	茯 苓
Semen Coicis Lachryma-jobi	Yi yi ren	薏 苡 仁
Rhizoma Atractylodis	Cang zhu	蒼 朮
Radix Puerariae	Ge gen	葛 根
Cortex Magnoliae Officinalis	Hou po	厚 樸
Herba Agastaches seu Pogostemi	Hou xiang	藿 香
Massa Fermenta	Shen qu	神 曲
Radix Vladimiriae	Chuan mu xiang	川 木 香
Radix Angelicae	Bai zhi	白 芷
Semen Paphani Sativi	Lai fu zi	萊 菔 子
Fructus Oryzae Sativae Germinantus	Gu ya	谷 芽
Pericarpium Citri Erythrocarpae	Ju hong	桔 紅
Herba Menthae	Bo he	薄 荷
Rhizoma Gastrodiae Elatae	Tian ma	天 麻
Flos Chrysanthemi Morifolii	Ju hua	菊 花

Eight Immortals Formula

INGREDIENTS

Radix Rehmanniae Glutinosae	Sheng di huang	生 地 黄
Tuber Ophiopogonis Japonici	Mai men dong	麥 門 冬
Herba Dendrobii	Shi hu	石 斛
Radix Dioscoreae Oppositae	Shan yao	山 藥
Fructus Corni Officinalis	Shan yu rou	山 萸 肉
Rhizoma Poly gonati Odorati	Yu zhu	玉 竹
Radix Adenophorae seu Glehniae	Sha shen	沙 參
Rhizoma Alismatis Plantago-aquaticae	Ze xie	澤 瀉
Cortex Moutan Radicis	Mu dan pi	牡 丹 皮
Poria	Fu ling	茯 苓
Fructus Schisandrae Chinensis	Wu wei zi	五 味 子

Essential Yang Formula

INGREDIENTS

Radix Rehmanniae Glutinosae	Sheng di huang	生 地 黄
Radix Dioscoreae Oppositae	Shan yao	山 藥
Fructus Lycii Chinensis	Gou qi zi	枸 杞 子
Radix Morindae Officinalis	Ba ji tian	巴 戟 天
Fructus Corni Officinalis	Shan yu rou	山 萸 肉
Herba Epimedii	Yin yang huo	淫 羊 藿
Rhizoma Alismatis Plantago-aquaticae	Ze xie	澤 瀉
Cortex Moutan Radicis	Mu dan pi	牡 丹 皮
Poria	Fu ling	茯 苓
Psoraleae Corylifoliae	Bu gu zhi	補 骨 脂
Cortex Cinnamomi Cassiae	Rou gui	肉 桂

Free and Easy Wanderer Plus

INGREDIENTS

Radix Bupleuri	Chai hu	柴 胡
Radix Angelicae Sinensis	Dang gui	當 歸
Radix Paeoniae Lactiflore	Bai shao	白 芍
Rhizoma Atractylodis Macrocephalae	Bai zhu	白 芷
Poria	Fu ling	茯 苓
Honey-toasted Radix Glycyrrhizae	Zhi gan cao	炙 甘 草
Radix Paeoniae Rubrae	Chi shao	赤 芍
Cortex Moutan Radicis	Mu dan pi	牡 丹 皮
Fructus Gardeniae Jasminoidis	Zhi zi	梔 子
Tuber Curcumae	Yu jin	郁 金
Herba Leonuri Heterophylli	Yi mu cao	益 母 草

Fritallaria and Pinellia Syrup

INGREDIENTS

Rhizoma Pinelliae Ternataae	Ban xia	半 夏
Bulbus Fritillariae Thunbergii	Zhe bei mu	浙 貝 母
Fructus Momordicae Grosvenori	Luo han guo	羅 漢 果
Herba Houttuyniae Cordatae	Yu xing cao	魚 腥 草
Concretio Silicea Bambusae	Tian zhu huang	天 竹 黄
Radix Scutellariae Baicalensis	Huang qin	黄 芩
Pericarpium Citri Reticulatae	Chen pi	陳 皮
Semen Pruni Armeniacae	Xing ren	杏 仁
Fructus Citri seu Ponciri Immaturus	Zhi shi	枳 實
Poria	Fu ling	茯 苓
Radix Glycyrrhizae Uralensis	Gan cao	甘 草

Gastrodis and Uncaria Formula

INGREDIENTS

Caulis Polygoni Multiflori	Ye jiao teng	夜交藤
Concha Haliotidis	Shi jue ming	石决明
Ramulus Loranthi	Sang ji sheng	桑寄生
Ramulus Uncariae Cum Uncis	Gou teng	鉤藤
Sclerotium Poriae Cocos Pararadicis	Fu shen	茯神
Radix Cyathulae	Chuan niu xi	川牛膝
Rhizoma Alismatis Plantago-aquticae	Ze xie	澤瀉
Rhizoma Gastrodiae Elatae	Tian ma	天麻
Fructus Gardeniae Jasminoidis	Zhi zi	枳子
Radix Scutellariae Baicalensis	Huang qin	黃芩
Herba Leonuri Heterophylli	Yi mu cao	益母草
Cortex Eucommiae Ulmidis	Du zhong	杜仲

General Tonic Formula

INGREDIENTS

Radix Codonopsis Pilosulae	Dang shen	黨參
Radix Rehmanniae Conquitae	Shu di huang	熟地黃
Radix Paeoniae Lactiflorae	Bai shao	白芍
Radix Angelicae Sinensis	Dang gui	當歸
Poria	Fu ling	茯苓
Rhizoma Atractylodis Macrocephalae	Bai zhu	白朮
Radix Astragali Membrannaceus	Huang qi	黃耆
Fructus Zizyphi Jujubae	Da zao	大棗
Radix Ligustici Chuanxiong	Chuan xiong	川芎
Radix Glycyrrhizae Uralensis	Gan cao	甘草
Cortex Einnamomi Cassiae	Rou gui	肉桂
Rhizoma Zingiberis Officinalis	Gan jiang	乾姜

Gentiana Drain Fire Formula

INGREDIENTS

Radix Rehmanniae Glutinosae	Sheng di huang	生地黄
Radix Scutellariae Baicalensis	Huang qin	黄耆
Fructus Gardeniae Jasminoidis	Zhi zi	枳子
Semen Plantaginis	Che qian zi	車前子
Rhizoma Alismatis Plantago-aquaticae	Ze xie	澤瀉
Radix Angelicae Sinensis	Dang gui	當歸
Cortex Moutan Radicis	Mu dan pi	牡丹皮
Radix Gentianae Scabrae	Long dan cao	龍膽草
Radix Glycyrrhizae Uralensis	Gan cao	甘草
Caulis Mutong	Mu tong	木通
Rhizoma Coptidis	Huang lian	黄連

Ginseng and Astragalus Formula

INGREDIENTS

Radix Astragali	Huang qi	黄耆
Rhizoma Atractylodis Macrocephalae	Bai zhu	白术
Radix Bupleuri	Chai hu	柴胡
Radix Angelicae Sinensis	Dang gui	當歸
Radix Glycyrrhizae Uralensis	Gan cao	甘草
Pericarpium Citri Reticulatae	Chen pi	陳皮
Radix Shih Chu Ginseng	Ren shen	人參
Rhizoma Cimicifugae	Sheng ma	升麻
Rhizoma Zingibeeris Officinalis	Gan jiang	乾姜

Ginseng Nourishing Formula

INGREDIENTS

Radix Paeoniae Lactiflorae	Bai shao	白芍
Radix Angelicae Sinensisn	Dang gui	當歸
Pericarpium Citri Reticulatae	Chen pi	陳皮
Radix Astragli	Huang qi	黃耆
Cortex Cinnamomi Cassiae	Rou gui	肉桂
Radix Shih Chu Ginseng	Ren shen	人參
Toasted Radix Glycyrrhizae	Zhi gan cao	炙甘草
Fructus Ziziphi Jujubae	Da zao	大棗
Fructus Schisandra Chinensis	Wu wei zi	五味子
Sclerotium Poriae Cocos	Fu shen	茯神
Radix Rehmanniae Conquitae	Shu di huang	熟地黃
Radix Polygalae Tenuifoliae	Yuan zhi	遠志
Rhizoma Zingiberis Officinalis	Gan jiang	乾姜

Heavenly Emperor's Formula

INGREDIENTS

Radix Rehmanniae Glutinosae	Sheng di huang	生地黃
Radix Codonopsis Pilosulae	Dang shen	黨參
Tuber Asparagi Cochinchinensis	Tian men dong	天門冬
Tuber Ophiopogonis Japonici	Mai men dong	麥門冬
Radix Angelicae Sinensis	Dang gui	當歸
Fructus Schisandrae Chinensis	Wu wei zi	五味子
Semen Biotaae Orientalis	Bai zi ren	柏子仁
Semen Ziziphi Spinosae	Suan zao ren	酸棗仁
Radix Scrophulaeriae Ningpoensis	Xuan shen	玄參
Radix Salviae miltiorrhizae	Dan shen	丹參
Sclerotium Poriae Cocos	Fu shen	茯神
Radix Polygalae Tenuifoliae	Yuan zhi	遠志
Radix P;atycodi Grandiflori	Jie geng	桔梗

Jade Screen and Xanthium Formula

INGREDIENTS

Radix Astragali	Huang qi	黄耆
Rhizoma Atractylodis Macrocephalae	Bai zhu	白朮
Radix Ledebouriellae Sesloidis	Fang feng	防風
Radix Paeoniae Rubra	Chi shao	赤芍
Fructus Forsythiae Suspensae	Lian qiao	連翹
Fructus Xanthii	Cang er zi	蒼耳子
Flos Magnoliae	Xin yi	辛荑
Radix Angelicae	Bai zhi	白芷

Juan Bi Formula

INGREDIENTS

Rhizoma et Radix Notopterygii	Qiang huo	羌活
Rhizoma Curcumae	Jiang huang	姜黄
Ramulus Mori Albae	Sang zhi	桑枝
Radix Angelicae	Dang gui	當歸
Radix Clematidis	Wei ling xian	威靈仙
Radix Duhuo	Du huo	獨活
Radix Gentianae Macrophylla	Qin jiao	秦艽
Gummi Olibanum	Ru xiang	乳香
Radix Aucklandiae Lappae	Mu xiang	木香
Radix Ligustici Chuanxiong	Chuan xiong	川芎
Raumlus Cinnamomi Cassiae	Gui zhi	桂枝
Honey-toasted Radix Glycyrrhizae Uralensis	Zhi gan cao	炙甘草

Lily Preserve Metal Formula

INGREDIENTS

Bulbus Lilii	Bai he	百合
Radix Rehmanniae Conquitae	Shu di huang	熟地黄
Radix Rehmanniae Glutinosae	Sheng di huang	生地黄
Radix Panacis Quinquefolii	Xi yang sheng	西洋參
Tuber Ophiopogonis Japonici	Mai men dong	麥門冬
Bulbus Fritillariae Cirrhosae	Chuan bei mu	川貝母

INGREDIENTS CONTINUED FROM PAGE 168

Radix Angelicae Sinensis	Dang gui	當歸
Radix Paeoniae Lactiflorae	Bai shao	白芍
Radix Glycyrrhizae Uralensis	Gan cao	甘草
Radix Scrophulariae Ningpoensis	Xuan shen	玄參
Radix Platycodi Grandiflori	Jie geng	桔梗

Ming Mu Formula

INGREDIENTS

Radix Rehmanniae Glutinosae Conquitae	Shu di huang	熟地黃
Radix Bupleuri	Chai hu	柴胡
Radix Angelicae Sinensis	Dang gui	當歸
Fructus Lycii	Gou qi zi	枸杞子
Radix Rehmanniae Glutinosae	Sheng di huang	生地黃
Radix Dioscoreae Oppositae	Shan yao	山藥
Fructus Comi Officinalis	Shan yu rou	山萸肉
Rhizoma Alismatis Plantago-aquaticae	Ze xie	澤瀉
Cortex Moutan Radicis	Mu dan pi	牡丹皮
Poria	Fu ling	茯苓
Fructus Schisandrae Chinensis	Wu wei zi	五味子
Fructus Tribuli Terrestris	Bai ji li	白蒺藜
Flos Chrysanthemi Morifolii	Bai ju hua	白菊花

Minor Bluegreen Dragon Formula

INGREDIENTS

Herba Asari cum Radice	Xi xin	細辛
Rhizoma Pinelliae Ternatae	Ban xia	半夏
Herba Ephedrae	Ma huang	麻黃
Ramulus Cinnmomi Cassiae	Gui zhi	桂枝
Rhizoma Zingiberis Officinalis	Sheng jiang	生姜
Fructus Schisandrae Chinensis	Wu wei zi	五味子
Radix Paeoniae Rubra	Chi shao	赤芍
Honey-toasted Radix Glycyrrhizae	Zhi gan cao	炙甘草
Radix Ledebouiellae Sesloidis	Fang feng	防風

Nourish Essence Formula

INGREDIENTS

Radix Rehmanniae	Shu di huang	熟 地 黄
Radix Dioscoreae	Sheng di huang	生 地 黄
Radix Polygoni Multiflori	He shou wu	何 首 烏
Fructus Corni	Shan zhu yu	山 茱 萸
Poria	Fu ling	茯 苓
Fructus Rubi	Fu pen zi	覆 盆 子
Semen Cuscutae	Tu si zi	兎 絲 子
Fructus Lycii Chinensis	Gou qi zi	枸 杞 子
Cortex Moutan Radicis	Mu dan pi	牡 丹 皮
Fructus Schisandrae	Wu wei zi	五 味 子
Herba Cistancher	Rou cong rong	肉 蓯 蓉
Rhizoma Alismatis	Ze xie	澤 瀉
Herba Cynomorii Songaricii	Suo yang	鎖 陽
Mel	Feng mi	蜂 蜜

Peaceful Spirit Formula

INGREDIENTS

Radix Codonopsis Pilosulae	Dang shen	黨 參
Fructus Ziziphi Jujubae	Da zao	大 棗
Radix Dioscoreae Oppositae	Shan yao	山 藥
Arillus Euphoriae Longanae	Long yan rou	龍 眼 肉
Radix Salviae Miltiorrhizae	Dan shen	丹 參
Sclerotium Poriae Cocos	Fu shen	茯 神
Radix Polygalae Tenuifoliae	Yuan zhi	遠 志
Radix Ginseng	Ren shen	人 參
Rhizoma Atractylodis Macrocephalae	Bai zhu	白 朮
Semen Ziziphi Spinosae	Suan zao ren	酸 棗 仁
Pericarpium Citri Reticulatae	Chen pi	陳 皮
Rhizoma Acori Garaminei	Shi chang pu	石 菖 蒲

Poria 15 Formula

INGREDIENTS

Semen Cassiae Torae	Jue ming zi	決 明 子
Rhizoma Alismatis Plantago-aquaticae	Ze xie	澤 瀉
Rhizoma Atractylodis Macrocephalae	Bai zhu	白 朮
Poria	Fu ling	茯 苓
Ramulus Cinnamomi Cassiae	Gui zhi	桂 枝
Fructus Citri seu Ponciri Immaturus	Zhi shi	枳 實
Fructus Crataegi	Shan zha	山 楂
Rhizoma Rhei	Da huang	大 黄
Semen Raphani Sativi	Lai fu zi	萊 菔 子
Herba Cistanches	Rou cong rong	肉 蓯 蓉
Radix Glycyrrhizae Uralensis	Gan cao	甘 草
Radix Vla dimiriae	Chuan mu xiang	川 木 香
Semen Pharbitidis	Qian niu zi	牽 牛 子
Radix Stephaniae Tetrandrae	Han fang ji	漢 防 己

Rehmannia and Scrophularia Formula

INGREDIENTS

Cortex phellodendri	Huang bai	黄 柏
Radix Anemarrhenae Asphodeloidis	Zhi mu	知 母

Salvia 10 Formula

INGREDIENTS

Radix Salviae Miltiorrhizae	Dan shen	丹 參
Tuber Curcumae	Yu jin	郁 金
Radix Paeoniae Rubra	Chi shao	赤 芍
Flos Albizziae Julibrissin	He huan hua	合 歡 皮
Radix Codonopsis Pilosulae	Dang shen	黨 參
Poria	Fu ling	茯 苓
Rhizoma Atractylodis Macrocephalae	Bai zhu	白 朮
Pericarpium Citri Reticulatae	Chen pi	陳 皮
Glycyrrhizae Uralensis	Gan cao	甘 草
Rhizoma Pinelliae Ternatae	Ban xia	半 夏

San Qi Tablets

INGREDIENTS

Radix Pseudoginseng	San qi	三七

Six Gentlemen Formula

INGREDIENTS SAME AS PROSPEROUS FARMER

Tang Kuei and Salvia Formula

INGREDIENTS

Radix Rehmanniae Glutinosae	Shu di huang	熟地黃
Radix Paeoniae Lactiflorae	Bai shao	白芍
Radix Polygoni Multiflori	He shou wu	何首烏
Radix Angelicae Sinensis	Dang gui	當歸
Radix Salviae Miltiorrhizae	Dan shen	丹參
Radix Ligustici Wallichii	Chuang xiong	川芎

Viola Clear Fire Formula

INGREDIENTS

Herba Oldenlandiae Diffusae	Bai hua she she cao	白花蛇舌草
Herba Houttuyniae Cordatae	Yu xing cao	魚腥草
Herba Violae cum Radice	Zi hua di ding	紫花地丁
Folium Daqingye	Da qing ye	大青葉
Radix Isatidis seu Baphicacanthi	Ban lan gen	板蘭根
Spica Prunellae Vulgaris	Xia ku cao	夏枯草
Herba Andrographis Paniculatae	Chuan xin lian	穿心蓮
Pericarpium Citri Reticulatae	Chen pi	陳皮
Flos Lonicerae Japonicae	Jin yin hua	金銀花
Fructus Forsythiae	Lian qiao	連翹
Usnea Longissima Ach.		
Radix Glycyrrhizae Uralensis	Gan cao	甘草
Rhizoma Coptids	Huang lian	黃連
Radix Lithospermi seu Arnebiae	Zi cao	紫草
Hypericum Perforatum		

Wu Hua Formula

INGREDIENTS

Flos Lonicerae Japonicae	Jin yin hua	金 銀 花
Flos Hibisci	Mu jin hua	木 槿 花
Flos Celosiae	Ji guan hua	雞 冠 花
Flos Magnoliae	Hou po hua	厚 樸 花
Flos Puerariae	Ge hua	葛 花

HEALTH CONCERNS

Adrenosen

INGREDIENTS

Dioscorea villosa		
L-phenylalanine		
Hypoxanthine riboside		
Pyridoxal alpha Ketoglutarate		
Radix Dioscoreae Oppositae	Shan yao	山 藥
Radix Pseudostellariae Heterophyllae	Tai zi shen	太 子 參
Fructus Schisandrae Chinensis	Wu wei zi	五 味 子
Semen Dolichoris Lablab	Bian dou	扁 豆
Fructus Oryzae Sativae Germinantus	Gu ya	谷 芽
Fructus Hordei Vulgaris Germinantus	Mai ya	麥 芽

Akebia Moist Heat Formula

INGREDIENTS SAME AS LOWER BURNER FORMULA

Aquilaria 22

INGREDIENTS

Lignum Aquilariae	Chen xiang	沉 香
Rhizoma Zingiberis Officinalis	Gan jiang	乾 姜
Fructus Pruni mume	Wu mei	烏 梅
Radix Codonopsis	Dang shen	黨 參
Fructus Terminaliae Chebulae	He zi	訶 子
Sclerotium Poriae Cocos	Fu ling	茯 苓
Rhizoma Atractylodis Macrocephalae	Bai zhu	白 朮
Fructus Quisqualis Indicae	Shi jun zi	使 君 子
Sclerotium Omphaliae Lapidescens	Lei wan	雷 丸
Radix Aucklandiae Lappae	Mu xiang	木 香
Semen Torreyae Grandis	Fei zi	榧 子
Pericarpium Punicae Granati	Shi liu pi	石 榴 皮
Fructus Meliae Toosendan	Chuan lian zi	川 楝 子
Fructus Rubi Chingii	Fu pen zi	覆 盆 子
Fructus Immaturus Citri Aurantii	Zhi shi	枳 實
Semen Myristicae Fragrantis	Rou dou kou	肉 豆 蔻
Semen Amomi Kravanh	Bai dou kou	白 豆 蔻
Fructus Evodiae	Wu yu	吳 萸
Pericarpium Zanthoxyli Bungeani	Hua jiao	花 椒
Radix Glycyrrhizae Uralensis	Gan cao	甘 草
Herba Aloes	Lu hui	蘆 薈

Astestatin

INGREDIENTS

Herba Artemisiae Annuae	Qing hao	青 蒿
Radix Dichroae Febrifugae	Chang shan	常 山
Radix Pulsatillae Chinensis	Bai tou weng	白 頭 翁
Cortex Magnoliae Officinalis	Hou po	厚 樸
Fructus Brucae Javanicae	Ya dan zi	鴉 膽 子
Rhizoma Pinelliae Ternatae	Ban xia	半 夏
Herba Agastaches seu Pogostemi	Huo xiang	藿 香
Semen Dolichoris Lablab	Bai bian dou	白 扁 豆

INGREDIENTS CONTINUED FROM PAGE 174

Radix Ginseng	Ren shen	人 參
Pericarpium Ctri Reticulatae	Chen pi	陳 皮
Radix Glycyrrhizae Uralensis	Gan cao	甘 草
Rhizoma Coptidis	Huang lian	黃 連
Rhizoma Atractylodis	Cang zhu	蒼 朮
Rhizoma Zingiberis Officinalis	Gan jiang	乾 姜
Fructus Amomi	Sha ren	砂 仁

New Astra 18 Diet

INGREDIENTS

Radix Astraguli Membranacei	Huang Qi	黃 耆
Rhizoma Alismatis Orientalis	Ze xie	澤 瀉
Fructus Gardeniae Jasminoidis	Zhi zi	梔 子
Rhizoma Cyperi Rotundi	Xiang fu zi	香 附 子
Radix Stephaniae Tetrandrae	Han fang ji	漢 防 己
Radix Angelicae Sinensis	Dang gui	當 歸
Radix Paeoniae Lactiflorae	Bai shao	白 芍
Rhizoma Atractylodis Macrocephalae	Bai zhu	白 朮
Radix Platycodi Grandiflori	Jie geng	桔 梗
Herba Sargassii	Hai zao	海 藻
Fructus Crataegi	Shan zha	山 楂
Radix Scutellariae Baicalensis	Huang qin	黃 芩
Rhizoma Zingiberis Officinalis	Gan jiang	乾 姜
Thallus Algae	Kun bu	昆 布
Cortex Magnoliae Officinalis	Hou po	厚 樸
Rhizoma Pinelliae Ternatae	Ban xia	半 夏
Pericarpium Citri Reticulatae	Chen pi	陳 皮

New Astra 8

INGREDIENTS

Radix Astragali Membranacei	Huang qi	黃耆
Fructus Arctii Lappae	Nu Zhen zi	女貞子
Excrementum Trogopteri seu Pteromi	Wu ling zhi	五靈脂
Radix Codonopsitis Pilosulae	Dang shen	黨參
Fructus Schisandrae Chinensis	Wu wei zi	五味子
Radix Glycyrrhizae Uralensis	Gan cao	甘草
Fructus Oryzae Sativae Germinantus	Gu ya	谷芽
Fructus Hordei Vulgaris Germinantus	Mai ya	麥芽
Eleutheroginseng	Wu jia shen	五加參

Astra C

INGREDIENTS

Vitamin C		
Radix Astraguli Membranacei	Huang qi	黃耆
Radix Atractylodis Macrocephalae	Bai zhu	白朮
Radix Ledebouriellae Divaricatae	Fang feng	防風
Zinc Citrate		
Rose Hips		
Acerola		

Astra Diet Tea

INGREDIENTS

Herba Menthae Haplocalycis	Bo he	薄荷
Eleutheroginseng	Wu jia shen	五加參
Rhizoma Zingiberis Officinalis	Gan jiang	乾姜
Folium Eriobotryae Japonicae	Pi pa ye	枇杷葉
Folium Perillae Frutescentis	Zi su ye	紫蘇葉

Astra Essence

INGREDIENTS

Radix Astraguli Membranacei	Huang qi	黃耆
Semen Astraguli Complanati	Sha yuan ji zi	沙苑蒺子
Fructus Ligustri Lucidi	Nu zhen zi	女貞子
Radix Polygoni Multiflori	He shou wu	何首烏
Fructus Lycii	Gou qi zi	枸杞子
Cortex Eucommiae Ulmoidis	Du zhong	杜仲
Semen Cuscutae Chinensis	Tu si zi	兎絲子
Radix Ginseng	Ren shen	人參
Radix Angelicae Sinensis	Dang gui	當歸
Fructus Corni Officinalis	Shan zhu yu	山茱萸

Astra Isatis

INGREDIENTS

Folium Daqingye	Da qing ye	大青葉
Radix Isatidis seu Baphicacanthi	Ban lan gen	板蘭根
Radix Astrguli Membranacei	Huang qi	黃耆
Radix Bupleuri	Chai hu	柴胡
Thallus Algae	Kun bu	昆布
Radix Codonopsitis Pilosulae	Dang shen	黨參
Radix et Rhizoma Polygoni Cuspidati	Yin yang huo	淫羊藿
Fructus Lycii	Gou qi zi	枸杞子
Radix Dioscoreae Oppositae	Shan yao	山藥
Radix Atractylodis Macrocephalae	Bai zhu	白朮
Radix Glycyrrhizae Uralensis	Gan cao	甘草
Halloysitum Rubrum	Chi shi zhi	赤石脂

Astrodia Relieve Wind Formula

INGREDIENTS

Rhizoma Gastrodiae Elatae	Tian ma	天 麻
Ramulus Uncariae cum Uncis	Gou teng	鉤 藤
Concha Haliotidis	Shi jue ming	石 決 明
Fructus Gardeniae Jasminoidis	Zhi zi	梔 子
Radix Scutellariae Baicalensis	Huang qin	黃 芩
Herba Leonuri Heterophylli	Yi mu cao	益 母 草
Radix Cyathulae Officinalis	Chuan niu xi	川 牛 膝
Cortex Eucommiae Ulmoidis	Du zhong	杜 仲
Ramulus Sangjusheng	Sang ju sheng	桑 寄 生
Caulis Polygoni Multiflori	Ye jiao teng	夜 交 藤
Sclerotium Poriae Cocos Rararadicis	Fu shen	茯 神

Bupleurum Entangles Qi Formula

INGREDIENTS

Radix Bulpleuri	Chai hu	柴 胡
Radix Angelicae Sinensis	Dang gui	當 歸
Cortex Fraxini	Qing pi	青 皮
Spica Prunellae Vulgaris	Xia ku cao	夏 枯 草
Radix Salviae Miltiorrhizae	Dan shen	丹 參
Radix Trichosanthis Kirilowii	Tian hua fen	天 花 粉
Semen Vaccariae Segetalis	Wang bu liu xing	王 不 留 行
Radix Paeoniae Lactiflorae	Bai shao	白 芍
Rhizoma Cyperi Rotundi	Xiang fu	香 附
Radix Ligustici Chuanxiong	Chuan xiong	川 芎
Bulbus Fritillariae Cirrhosae	Chuan bei mu	川 貝 母
Herba Taraxaci Mongolici cum Radice	Pu gong ying	蒲 公 英
Radix Paeoniae Rubrae	Chi shao	赤 芍

Calm Spirit

INGREDIENTS

Enzymes: 300 mg
Horseradish root
Aspergillus niger
Aspergillus oryzae (Amylase, Protease, Lipease)
Taurine: 100 mg
Calcined Magnetite asparatate

Semen Biotae Orientalis	Bai zhi ren	柏智仁
Radix Angelicae Sinensis	Dang gui	當歸
Sclerotium Poriae Cocos Pararadicis	Fu shen	茯神
Radix Polygalae Tenuifoliae	Yuan zhi	遠志
Semen Zizyphi Spinosae	Suan zao ren	酸棗仁
Radix Paeoniae Lactiflorae	Bai shao	白芍
Tuber Ophiopogonis Japonici	Mai men dong	麥門冬
Radix Codonopsitis Pilosulae	Dang shen	黨參
Succinum	Hu po	琥珀

Clear Heat

INGREDIENTS

Radix Istidis seu Baphicacanthi	Ban lan gen	板蘭根
Folium Daqingye	Da qing ye	大青葉
Herba Hedyotidis Diffusae	Bai hua she she cao	白花蛇舌草
Flos Lonicerae Japonicae	Jin yin hua	金銀花
Spica Prunellae Vulgaris	Xia ku cao	夏枯草
Herba Andrographitis Paniculatae	Chuan xin lian	穿心蓮
Thallus Algae	Kun bu	昆布
Herba cum Radice Violae Yedoensitis	Zi hua di ding	紫花地丁
Cordyceps Sinensis	Dong chong xia cao	冬蟲夏草
Radix Glycyrrhizae Uralensis	Gan cao	甘草

Clearing

INGREDIENTS

Semen Nelumbinis Nuciferae	Lian zi	蓮 子
Tuber Ophiopogonis Japonici	Mai men dong	麥 門 冬
Sclerotium Poriae Cocos	Fu ling	茯 苓
Radix Ginseng	Ji lin shen	吉 林 參
Semen Plantaginis	Che qian zi	車 前 草
Radix Scutellariae Baicalensis	Huang qin	黃 芩
Herba Dendrobii	Shi hu	石 斛
Rhizoma Smilacis Glabrae	Tu fu ling	土 茯 苓
Radix Astraguli Membranacei	Huang qi	黃 耆
Cortex Lycii Radicis	Di gu pi	地 骨 皮
Cortex Moutan Radicis	Mu dan pi	牡 丹 皮
Radix Paeoniae Rubrae	Chi shao	赤 芍
Radix Glycyrrhi Uralensis	Gan cao	甘 草

Clear Phlegm

INGREDIENTS

Rhizoma Pinelliae Ternatae	Ban xia	半 夏
Pericarpium Citri Reticulatae	Chen pi	陳 皮
Sclerotium Poriae Cocos	Fu ling	茯 苓
Fructus Immaturus Citri Aurantii	Zhi shi	枳 實
Caulis Bambusae in Taeniis	Zhu ru	竹 茹
Rhizoma Arisaematis	Tian nan xing	天 南 星
Herba Agastaches seu Pogostemi	Huo xiang	藿 香
Rhizoma Acori Graminei	Shi chang pu	石 菖 蒲
Radix Glycyrrhi Uralensis	Gan cao	甘 草

Colostroplex

INGREDIENTS

Bovine Colostrum Complex

Coptis Purge Fire Formula

INGREDIENTS

Rhizoma Coptidis	Huang lian	黄 連
Herba Lophatheri Gracilis	Dan zhu ye	淡 竹 葉
Radix Bupleuri	Chai hu	柴 胡
Rehmanriae Glutinose	Sheng di huang	生 地 黄
Radix Angelicae Sinensis	Dang gui	當 歸
Radix Paeoniaae Lactiflorae	Bai shao	白 芍
Rhizoma Anemarrhenae Asphodeloidis	Zhi mu	知 母
Caulis Clematidis Armandii	Mu tong	木 通
Radix Scutillariae Baicalensis	Huang qin	黄 芩
Cortex Phelloodendri	Huang bai	黄 柏
Rhizoma Alismatis Orientalis	Ze xie	澤 瀉
Semen Plantaginis	Che qian zi	車 前 子
Radix Gentianae Longdancao	Long dan cao	龍 膽 草
Fructus Forsythiae Suspensae	Lian qiao	連 翹
Fructus Gardeniae Jasminoidis	Zhi zi	梔 子
Radix Glycyrrhizae Uralensis	Gan cao	甘 草
Radix Sophorae Flavescentis	Ku shen	苦 參

Crampbark Plus

INGREDIENTS

Viburnum Opulis Crampbark		
Ramulus Cinnamomi Cassiae	Gui zhi	桂 枝
Radix Achyranthis Bidentatae	Niu xi	牛 膝
Radix Paeoniae Rubrae	Chi shao	赤 芍
Cortex Moutan Radiicis	Mu dan pi	牡 丹 皮
Herba Leonuri Heterophylli	Yi mu cao	益 母 草
Rhizoma Corydalis Yanhusuo	Yan hu suo	延 胡 索
Radix Angelicae Sinensis	Dang gui	當 歸
Semsn Persicae	Tao ren	桃 仁
Rhizoma Curcumae Ezhu	E zhu	莪 朮
Rhizoma Sparganii Stoloniferi	San leng	三 稜
Rhizoma Cyperi Rotundi	Xiang fu	香 附
Radix Aucklandiae Lappae	Mu xiang	木 香
Flos Carthami Tinctorii	Hong hua	紅 花

Drain Dampness

INGREDIENTS

Rhizoma Alismatis	Ze xie	澤 瀉
Sclerotium Poriae Cocos	Fu ling	茯 苓
Sclerotium Poly Umbellati	Zhu ling	豬 苓
Ramulus Cinnamomi Cassiae	Gui zhi	桂 枝
Rhizoma Atractylodis Macrocephalae	Bai zhu	白 朮

Ease Plus

INGREDIENTS

Concha Ostreae	Mu li	牡 蠣
Os Draconis	Long gu	龍 骨
Radix Bupleuri	Chai hu	柴 胡
Radix Ginseng	Ren shen	人 參
Rhizoma Zingiberis Officinalis	Gan jiang	乾 姜
Rhizoma Pinelliae Ternatae	Ban xia	半 夏
Radix Scutellariae Baicalensis	Huang qin	黃 芩
Ramulus Cinnamomi Cassiae	Gui zhi	桂 枝
Radix et Rhizoma Rhei	Da huang	大 黃
Radix Aucklandiae Lappae	Mu xiang	木 香

Eight Treasures

INGREDIENTS

Radix Codonopsitis Pilosulae	Dang shen	黨 參
Rhizoma Atractylodis Macrocephalae	Bai zhu	白 朮
Sclerotium Poriae Cocos	Fu ling	茯 苓
Radix Rehmanniae Glutinosae Conquitae	Shu di huang	熟 地 黃
Radix Paeoniae Lactiflorae	Bai shao	白 芍
Fructus Zizyphi Jujubae	Da zao	大 棗
Radix Angelicae Sinensis	Dang gui	當 歸
Radix Ligustici Chanuxiong	Chuan xiong	川 芎
Radix et Caulis Jixueteng	Ji xue teng	雞 血 藤
Radix Glycyrrhizae Uralensis	Zhi gan cao	炙 甘 草
Rhizoma Zingiberis Officinalis	Gan jiang	乾 姜

Essence Chamber

INGREDIENTS

Serronoae Serrulatae		
Radix Salviae Miltiorrhizae	Dan shen	丹 參
Semen Vaccariae Segetalis	Wang bu liu xing	王 不 留 行
Fructus Liquidambaris Taiwanianae	Lu lu tong	路 路 通
Hyfrangeae arborscentis		
Turnerae aphrodisiacae		
Sclerotium Poriae Cocos	Fu ling	茯 苓
Rhizoma Dioscoreae Hypogloaucae	Bei xie	萆 薢
Semen Benincasae Hispidae	Dong gua zi	冬 瓜 子

Fertile Garden

INGREDIENTS

Ramulus Sangjisheng	Sang ji sheng	桑 寄 生
Fructus Ligustri Licidi	Nu zhen zi	女 貞 子
Fructus Amomi	Sha ren	砂 仁
Semen Cuscutae Chinensis	Tu si zi	兎 絲 子
Radix Pseudostellariae Heterophyllae	Tai zi shen	太 子 參
Tuber Asparagi Cochinchinensis	Tian men dong	天 門 冬
Radix Angelicae Sinensis	Dang gui	當 歸
Radix Paeoniae Lactiflorae	Bai shao	白 芍
Fructus Lycii	Gou qi zi	枸 杞 子
Sclerotium Poriae Cocos	Fu ling	茯 苓
Fructus Meliae Toosendan	Chuan lian zi	川 楝 子
Radix Glycyrrhizae Uralensis	Zhi gan cao	炙 甘 草
Placenta Hominis	Zi he che	紫 河 車
Awithaniae somniferae		
Helonias diocia		

Flabonex

INGREDIENTS

Radix Puerariae	Ge gen	葛 根
Ilex Pubescens Hook. Et Arn	Mao dong qing	毛 冬 青
Radix Salviae Miltiorrhizae	Dan shen	丹 參
Flos Lonicerae Japonicae	Jin yin hua	金 銀 花
Cortex Eucommiae Ulmoidis	Du zhong	杜 仲
Cistanches Deserticolae	Rou cong rong	肉 蓯 蓉
Radix Polygoni Mnultiflori	He shou wu	何 首 烏
Fructus Mori Albae	Sang shen	桑 椹
Fructus Rosae Laevigatae	Jin ying zi	金 櫻 子
Fructus Lycii	Gou qi zi	枸 杞 子
Semen Zizyphi Spinosae	Suan zao ren	酸 棗 仁
Radix Angelicae Sinensis	Dang gui	當 歸
Fructus Schisandrae Chinensis	Wu wei zi	五 味 子
Folium Ginkgo Bilobae	Bai guo ye	白 果 葉

Formula H

INGREDIENTS

Radix Pulsatillae Chinensis	Bai tou weng	白 頭 翁
Flos Sophorae Japonicae Immaturus	Huai hua mi	槐 花 米
Radix Paeoniae Lactiflorae	Bai shao	白 芍
Radix Angelicae Sinensis	Dang gui	當 歸
Drosera	Jin di luo	金 地 落
Flos Lonicerae Japonicae	Jin yin hua	金 銀 花
Radix Sanguisorbae Officinalis	Di yu	地 榆
Radix Rehmanniae Glutinosae	Sheng di huang	生 地 黄
Cortex Fraxini	Qin pi	秦 皮
Cortex Phellodendri	Huang bai	黄 柏

Gentle Senna

INGREDIENTS

Microcos Pariculata	Po bu ye	破布葉
Flos Lonicerae Japonicae	Jin yin hua	金銀花
Folium Sennae	Fan xie ye	番瀉葉
Semen Pruni	Yu li ren	郁李仁
Flos Radicis Puerariae	Ge hua	葛花
Semen Arecae Catechu	Bing lang	檳榔

Ginseng and Gecko Herbal Formula

INGREDIENTS

Semen Pruni Armeniacae	Ku xing ren	苦杏仁
Radix Glycyrrhizae Uralensis	Zhi gan cao	炙甘草
Radix Ginseng	Ren shen	人參
Sclerotium Poriae Cocos	Fu ling	茯苓
Cortex Mori Albae Radicis	Sang bai pi	桑白皮
Bulbus Fritillariae Cirrhosae	Chuan bei mu	川貝母
Rhizoma Anemarrhenae Asphodeloidis	Zhi mu	知母
Gecko	Ge jie	蛤蚧

Head-Q

INGREDIENTS

Flos Chrysanthemi Morifolii	Ju hua	菊花
Rhizoma et Radix Notopterygii	Qiang huo	羌活
Tuber Ophiopogonis Japonici	Mai men dong	麥門冬
Rhizoma Atractylodis Macrocephalae	Bai zhi	白芷
Radix Ligustici Chuanxiong	Chuan xiong	川芎
Radix Ledebouriellae Divaricatae	Fang feng	防風
Radix Scutellariae Baicalensis	Huang qin	黄芩
Radix Angelicae Sinensis	Dang gui	當歸
Rhizoma Zingiberis Officinalis	Gan jiang	乾姜
Herba cum Raice Asari	Xi xin	細辛
Radix Rehmanniae Glutinosae	Sheng di huang	生地黄
Fructus Viticis	Man jing zi	蔓荆子
Rhizoma et Radix Ligustici	Gao ben	藁本
Western Chrysanthenum		

Isatis Cooling Formula

INGREDIENTS

Radix Isatidis seu Baphicacanthi	Ban lan gen	板 蘭 根
Folium Daqingye	Da qing ye	大 青 葉
Radix Codonopsitis Pilosulae	Dang shen	黨 參
Concha Ostreae	Mu li	牡 蠣
Radix Bupleuri	Chai hu	柴 胡
Rhizoma Smilacis Glabrae	Tu fu ling	土 茯 苓
Fructus Gardeniae Jasminoidis	Zhi zi	梔 子
Cortex Moutan Radicis	Mu dan pi	牡 丹 皮
Radix Angelicae Sinensis	Dang gui	當 歸
Caulis Mutong	Mu tong	木 通
Radix Paeoniae Rubrae	Chi shao	赤 芍
Rhizoma Alismatis Orientalis	Ze xie	澤 瀉
Rhizoma Cyperi Rotundi	Xiang fu	香 附

Isatis Gold

INGREDIENTS

Radix Isatidis seu Baphicacanthi	Ban lan gen	板 蘭 根
Folium Daqingye	Da qing ye	大 青 葉
Radix Platycodi Grandiflori	Jie geng	桔 梗
Radix Ligustici Chuanxiong	Chuan xiong	川 芎
Echinacea purpura		
Hydrastic canadensis		

Jin Qian Cao Stone Formula

INGREDIENTS

Herba Lysimachiae	Jin qian cao	金 錢 草
Spora Lygodii Japonici	Hai jin sha	海 金 沙
Radix Bupleuri	Chai hu	柴 胡
Semen Plantaginis	Che qian zi	車 前 子
Herba Polygoni Avicularis	Bian xu	萹 蓄
Herba Dianthi	Qu mai	瞿 麥
Radix Paeoniae Rubrae	Chi shao	赤 芍
Fructus Gardeniae Jasminoidis	Zhi zi	梔 子
Herba Artemisiae Yinchenhao	Yin chen	茵 陳
Fructus Immaturus Citri Aurantii	Zhi shi	枳 實
Radix Notoginseng	San qi	三 七
Radix Glycyrrhizae Uralensis	Gan cao	甘 草

Marrow Plus

INGREDIENTS

Radix et Caulis Jixueteng	Ji sue teng	雞 血 藤
Radix Polygoni Multiflori	He shou wu	何 首 烏
Radix Salviae Miltiorrhizae	Dan shen	丹 參
Radix Codonopsitis Pilosulae	Dang shen	黨 參
Radix Astroguli Membranacei	Huang qi	黃 耆
RhizomaLigustici Chuanxiong	Chuan xiong	川 芎
Radix Rehmanniae Glutinosae	Sheng di huang	生 地 黃
Radix Rehmanniae Glutinosae Conquitae	Shu di huang	熟 地 黃
Fructus Lycii	Gou qi zi	枸 杞 子
Radix Angelicae Sinensis	Dang gui	當 歸
Semen Nelumbinis Nuciferae	Lian zi	蓮 子
Pericarpium Citri Reticulatae	Chen pi	陳 皮
Fructus Zizyphi Jujubae	Da zao	大 棗
Fructus Oryzae Sativae Germinantus	Gu ya	谷 芽
Gelatinum Corii Asini	E jiao	阿 膠

Maternal Herbal

INGREDIENTS

Radix ginseng	Ji lin shen	吉 林 參
Cistanches Deserticolae	Rou cong rong	肉 蓯 蓉
Radix Rehmanniae Gluinosae Conquitae	Shu di huang	熟 地 黃
Radix Angelicae Sinensis	Dang gui	當 歸
Frucus Ligustri Lucidi	Nu zhen zi	女 貞 子
Fructus Rubi Chingii	Fu pen zi	覆 盆 子
Cornu Cervi Degelatinatium	Lu jiao jiao	鹿 角 膠
Radix Morindae Officinalis	Ba ji tian	巴 戟 天
Herba Cynomorii Songarici	Suo yang	鎖 陽
Sclerotium Poriae Cocos Pararadicis	Fu shen	茯 神
Radix Ligustici Chuanxiong	Chuan xiong	川 芎
Cortex Eucommiae Ulmoidis	Du zhong	杜 仲
Herba Epimedii	Yin yang huo	淫 羊 藿
Fructus Evodiae Rutaecarpae	Wu zhu yu	吳 茱 萸
Cortex Cinnamomi Cassiae	Rou gui	肉 桂
Pericarpium Zanthoxyli Bungeani	Chuan jiao	川 椒

Minor Blue Dragon

INGREDIENTS

Rhizoma Pinelliae Ternatae	Ban xia	半 夏
Radix Glycyrrhizae Uralensis	Gan cao	甘 草
Fructus Schisandrae Chinensis	Wu wei zi	五 味 子
Herba Ephedrae	Ma huang	麻 黃
Ramulus Cinnamomi Cassiae	Gui zhi	桂 枝
Rhizopma Zingiberis Officinalis	Gan jiang	乾 姜
Radix Paeoniae Lactiflorae	Bai shao	白 芍
Herba cum Radice Asari	Xi xin	細 辛

Mobility 2

INGREDIENTS

Radix Paeoniae Rubrae	Chi shao	赤 芍
Radix Angelicae Sinensis	Dang gui	當 歸
Radix Ligustice Chuan xiong	Chuan xiong	川 芎
Radix Rehmannia Glutinosae Conquitae	Shu di hunag	熟 地 黃
Semen Persicae	Tao ren	桃 仁
Radix Angelicae Dahuricae	Bai zhi	白 芷
Sclerotium Poriae Cocos	Fu ling	茯 苓
Radix Ledebouriellae Divaricatae	Fang feng	防 風
Pericarpium Citri Reticualatae	Chen pi	陳 皮
Radix Stephniae Tetrandrae	Fang ji	防 己
Radix Gentianae Qinjiao	Qin jiao	秦 艽
Rhizoma et Radix Notopterygii	Qiang huo	羌 活
Radix Clematidis	Wei ling xian	威 靈 仙
Rhizoma Zingiberis Officinalis	Gan jiang	乾 姜
Radix Angelicae Dahuricae	Bai zhi	白 芷
Radix Glycyrrhizae Uralensis	Gan cao	甘 草

Mobility 3

INGREDIENTS

Radix Ginseng	Ji lin shen	吉 林 參
Ramulus Cinnamomi Cassiae	Gui zhi	桂 枝
Radix Rehmanniae Glutinosae Conquitae	Shu di huang	熟 地 黃
Radix Polygoni Multiflori	He shou wu	何 首 烏
Ramulus Sangjisheng	Sang ji sheng	桑 寄 生
Rhiaoma et Radix Notopterygii	Qiang huo	羌 活
Radix Angelicae Sinensis	Dang gui	當 歸
Cistanches Deserticolae	Rou cong rong	肉 蓯 蓉
Ardisia Gigantifolia	Zou Ma tai	走 馬 胎
Radix Angelicae Pubescentis	Du huo	獨 活
Radix Notoginseng	San qi	三 七
Radix et Caulis Jixueteng	Ji xue teng	雞 血 藤
Herba cum Radice Asari	Xi xin	細 辛

INGREDIENTS CONTINUED FROM PAGE 189

Ramus tinosporae Sinensis	Shu jin teng	舒筋藤
Fructus Chaenomelis	Mu gua	木瓜
Radix Achyranthis Bidentatae	Niu xi	牛膝

Nasal Tab

INGREDIENTS

Radix Ephedrae	Ma huang	麻黄
Flos Magnoliae	Xin yi	辛荑
Radix Puerariae	Ge gen	葛根
Radix et Rhizoma Rhei	Da huang	大黄
Semen Coicis Lachryma-jobi	Yi yi ren	薏苡仁
Gypsum	Shi gao	石膏
Ramulus Cinnamomi Cassiae	Gui zhi	桂枝
Radix Paeoniae Rubrae	Chi shao	赤芍
Rhizoma Zingiveris Officinalis	Gan jiang	乾姜
Radix Glycyrrhizae Uralensis	Gan cao	甘草
Radix Ligustici Chuanxiong	Chuan xiong	川芎
Frtuctus Zizyphi Jujubae	Da zao	大棗
Radix Platycodi Grandiflori	Jie geng	桔梗

Nine Flavor Tea

INGREDIENTS

Radix Rehmanniae Glutinosae Conquitae	Shu di huang	熟地黄
Radix Rehmanniae Glutinasae	Sheng di huang	生地黄
Radix Dioscoreae Oppositae	Shan yao	山藥
Sclerotium Poriae Cocos	Fu ling	茯苓
Fructus Corni Officinalis	Shan zhu yu	山茱萸
Cortex Moutan Radicis	Mu dan pi	牡丹
Rhizoma Alismatis Orientalis	Ze xie	澤瀉
Herba Dendrobii	Shi hu	石斛
Radix Scrophulariae Ningpoensis	Xuan shen	玄參
Tuber Ophiopogonis Japonici	Mai men dong	麥門冬

Phellostatin

INGREDIENTS

Cortex Phellodendri	Huang bai	黄 柏
Radix Codonopsitis Rutaecarpae	Dang shen	黨 參
Rhizoma Atractylodis Macrocephalae	Bai zhu	白 朮
Rhizoma Anemarrhenae Asphodeloidis	Zhi mu	知 母
Semen Plantaginis	Che qian zi	車 前 子
Radix Pulsatillae Chinensis	Bai tou weng	白 頭 翁
Herba Artemisiae Yinchenhao	Yin chen hao	茵 陳 蒿
Fructus Cnidii Monnieri	She chuang zi	蛇 床 子
Herba cum Radice Houttuyniae Cordatae	Yu xing cao	魚 腥 草
Radix Dioscoreae Oppositae	Shan yao	山 藥
Radix Glycyrrhizae Uralensis	Gan cao	甘 草
Pericarpum Amomi	Sha ren ke	砂 仁 殼

Power Mushrooms

INGREDIENTS

Excrementum Trogopteri seu Pteromi	Wu ling zhi	五 靈 脂
Fructuficatio Tremellae Fuciformis	Bai mu er	白 木 耳
Sclerotium Poriae Cocos	Fu ling	茯 苓
Sclerotium Polypori Umbellari	Zhu ling	豬 苓

Quiet Digestion

INGREDIENTS

Sclerotium Poriae Cocos	Fu ling	茯 苓
Semen Coicis Lachryma-jobi	Yi yi ren	益 苡 仁
Massa Fermentata	Shen qu	神 曲
Cortex Magnoliae Officinalis	Hou po	厚 樸
Radix angelicae Dahuricae	Bai zhi	白 芷
Radix Puerariae	Ge gen	葛 根
Rhizoma Atractylodis	Cang zhu	蒼 朮
Radix Aucklandiae Lappae	Mu xiang	木 香
Herba Agastaches seu Pogostemi	Huo xiang	藿 香

INGREDIENTS CONTINUED FROM PAGE 191

Fructus Oryzae Sativae Germinantus	Gu ya	谷芽
Radix Trichosantis Kirilowii	Tian hua fen	天花粉
Flos Cheysanthemi Morifolii	Ju hua	菊花
Rubrum Halloysitum	Chi shi zhi	茨實子
Pars Rubra Epicarpii Citri Erythrocarpae	Ju hong	桔紅
Herba Menthae Haplocalycis	Bo he	薄荷

Rehmannia 8

INGREDIENTS SAME AS DYNAMIC WARRIOR

New Reinall K

INGREDIENTS

Sanguis Draconis	Xue jie	血竭
Pasta Acaciae seu Uncariae	Er cha	兒茶
Rhizoma Corydalis Yanhusuo	Yan hu suo	延胡索
Flos Carthami Tinctorii	Hong hua	紅花
Myrrha	Mo yao	沒藥
Gummi Olibanum	Ru xiang	乳香
Borneol	Bing pian	冰片
Alcohol		
Glycerin		
Piper methysticum		

Schizandra Dreams

INGREDIENTS

Piper Methysticum		
Fructus Schisandrae Chinensis	Wu wei zi	五味子
Concha Ostreae	Mu li	牡蠣
Os Draconis	Long gu	龍骨
Succinum	Hu po	琥珀

Shen-Gem

INGREDIENTS SAME AS GATHER VITALITY

Shu Gan

INGREDIENTS

Tuber Curcumae	Yu jin	郁 金
Lignum Aquilariae	Chen xiang	沉 香
Rhizoma Corydalis Yanhusuo	Yan hu suo	延 胡 索
Radix Aucklandiae Lappae	Mu xiang	木 香
Semen Myristicae Frangrantis	Rou dou kou	肉 豆 蔻
Radix Paeoniae Lactiflorae	Bai shao	白 芍
Fructus Citri Aurantii	Zhi ke	枳 殼
Pericarpium Citri Reticulatae	Chen pi	陳 皮
Fructus Amomi	Sha ren	砂 仁
Cortex Magnoliae Officinalis	Hou po	厚 樸
Rhizoma Cyperi Routundi	Xiang fu	香 附
Radix Glycyrrhizae Uralensis	Gan cao	甘 草
Cortex Moutan Radicis	Mu dan pi	牡 丹 皮
Pericarpium Citri Reticulatae Viride	Qing pi	青 皮
Lignum Santali Albi	Tan xiang	檀 香

Six Gentlemen

INGREDIENTS SAME AS PROSPEROUS FARMER

Skin Balance

INGREDIENTS

Herba Scutellariae Barbatae	Ban zhi lian	半 枝 蓮
Herba Hedyotidis Diffusae	Bai hau she she cao	白 花 蛇 舌 草
Radix Gentianae Lang dancao	Long dan cao	龍 膽 草
Radix Rehmanniae Glutinosae	Sheng di huang	生 地 黃
Herba cum Radice Violae Yedoensitis	Zi hua di ding	紫 花 地 丁
Radix Ledebouriellae Divaricatae	Fang feng	防 風

Flos Lonicerae Japonicae	Jin yin hua	金銀花
Herba Lygodii Japonici	Jin qian cao	金錢草
Rhizoma Coptidis	Huang lian	黃連
Radix Angelicae Sinensis	Dang gui	當歸
Radix Bupleuri	Chai hu	柴胡
Flos Carthami Tinctorii	Hong hua	紅花
Folium Senae	Fan xie ye	番瀉葉
Radix et Rhizoma	Da huang	大黃

Source Qi

INGREDIENTS

Cortex Ailanthi Altissimae	Chun pi	椿皮
Radix Astragali Membranalis	Huang qi	黃耆
Radix Ginseng	Ren shen	人參
Radix Angelicae Dahuricae	Bai zhi	白芷
Rhizoma Atractylodis	Cang zhu	蒼朮
Sclerotium Poriae Cocos	Fu ling	茯苓
Radix Dioscoreae Oppositae	Shan yao	山藥
Semen Nelumbinis Nuciferae	Lian rou	蓮肉
Semen Euryales Ferocis	Qian shi	芡實
Rhizoma Cimicifugae	Sheng ma	升麻
Rhizoma Zingiberis Officinalis	Gan jiang	乾姜
Radix Bupleuri	Chai hu	柴胡
Semen Myristicae Fragrantis	Rou dou kou	肉豆蔻
Radix Glycyrrhizae Uralensis	Zhi gan cao	炙甘草
Massa Fermentata	Shen qu	神曲

Stomach Tablets

INGREDIENTS

Cortex Magnoliae Officinalis	Hou po	厚樸
Pericarpium Citri Reticulatae	Chen pi	陳皮
Rhizoma Pineliae Ternatae	Ban xia	半夏
Rhizoma Atractylodis	Cang zhu	蒼朮

Rhizoma Zingiberis Officinalis	Gan jiang	乾 姜
Radix Glycyrrhizae Uralensis	Gan cao	甘 草
Radix Bupleuri	Chai hu	柴 胡
Fructus Oryzae Sativae Germinantus	Gu ya	谷 芽

Tremella and American Ginseng

INGREDIENTS

Fructificatio Tremellae Fuciformis	Bai mu er	白 木 耳
Radix Panacis Quinquefolii	Xi yang shen	西 洋 參
Radix Astragali Membranacei	Huang qi	黄 耆
Fructus Schisandrae Chinensis	Wu wei zi	五 味 子
Radix Rehmanniae Glutinosae	Sheng di huang	生 地 黃
Fructus Lycii	Gou qi zi	枸 杞 子
Cortex Lycii Radicis	Di gu pi	地 骨 皮
Radix Isatidis seu Baphicacanthi	Ban lan gen	板 蘭 根
Folium Daqingye	Da qing ye	大 青 葉
Tuber ophiopogonis Jponici	Mai men dong	麥 門 冬
Herba cum Radice Violae Yedoensitis	Zi hua di ding	紫 花 地 丁
Excrementum Trogopteri seu Pteromi	Wu ling zhi	五 靈 脂
Semen Cuscutae Chinensis	Tu si zi	兎 絲 子
Herba Dendrobii	Shi hu	石 斛
Radix et Caulis Jixueteng	Ji xue teng	雞 血 藤
Fructus Ligustri Lucidi	Nu zhen zi	女 貞 子
Radix Adenophorae seu Glehniae	Sha shen	沙 參
Radix Angelicae Sinensis	Dang gui	當 歸
Plastrum Testudinis	Gui ban	龜 板
Herba Epimedii	Yin yang huo	淫 羊 藿
Pericarpium Citri Reticulatae	Chen pi	陳 皮
Tuber Curcumae	Yu jin	郁 金
Radix Glycyrrhizae Uralensis	Gan cao	甘 草
Fructus Amomi	Sha ren	砂 仁

Two Immortals

INGREDIENTS

Fructus Schisandrae Chinensis	Wu wei zi	五味子
Concha Ostreae	Mu li	牡蠣
Herba Epimediii	Yin yang huo	淫羊藿
Radix Morindae Officinalis	Ba ji tian	巴戟天
Radix Angelicae Sinensis	Dang gui	當歸
Fructux Ligustri Lucidi	Nu zhen zi	女貞子
Herba Ecliptae Prostratae	Han lian cao	旱蓮草
Folium Turnerae Aphrodisiacae		
Radix Hydrocotyle Asiaticae		
Radix Pseudostellariae Heterophyllae	Tai zi shen	太子參
Fructus Zizyphi Jujubae	Da zao	大棗
Rhizoma Anemarrhenae Asphodeloidis	Zhi mu	知母
Corte Phellodendri	Huang bai	黃柏
Radix Glycyrrhizae Uralensis	Zhi gan cao	炙甘草
Radix Scrophulariae Ningpoensis	Xuan shen	玄參
Fructus Akebiae	Ba yue zha	八月扎

Unlocking Formula

INGREDIENTS

Herba cum Radice Patriniae	Bai jiang cao	敗醬草
Caulis Sargentodoxae Cuneatae	Da xue teng	大血藤
Radix Cyathulae Officinalis	Chuan niu xi	川牛膝
Fructus Meliae Toosendan	Chuan lian zi	川楝子
Cortex Moutan Radicis	Mu dan pi	牡丹皮
Radix Paeoniae Rubrae	Chi shao	赤芍
Sclerotium Poriae Cocos	Fu ling	茯苓
Fructus Foeniculi Vulgaris	Xiao hui xiang	小茴香
Semen Citri Reticulatae	Ju he	桔核
Rhizoma Atractylodis	Cang zhu	蒼朮
Rhizoma Atractylodis Macrocephalae	Bai zhu	白朮
Cortex Phellodendri	Huang bai	黃柏
Rhizoma Cimicifugae	Sheng ma	升麻

Virility Tabs

INGREDIENTS

Radix Ginseng	Ji lin shen	吉林參
Yu biao	Yu biao	魚鰾
Cistanches Deserticolae	Rou cong rong	肉蓯蓉
Radix Morindae Officinalis	Ba ji tian	巴戟天
Radix Astragali Membranacei	Huang qi	黃耆
Cornu Cervi Degelatinati	Lu jiao shuang	鹿角霜
Radix Dipsaci Asperi	Xu duan	續斷
Radix Angelicae Sinensis	Dang gui	當歸
Fructus Psoraleae Corylifoliae	Bu gu zhi	補骨脂
Cortex Eucommiae Ulmoidis	Du zhong	杜仲
Herba Cynomorii Songdici	Suo yang	鎖陽
Radix Rehmanniae Glutinosae Conquitae	Shu di huang	熟地黃
Fructus Amomi	Sha ren	砂仁
Gelatinum Corii Asini	E jiao	阿膠
Cortex Cinnamomi Cassiae	Rou gui	肉桂

Woman's Balance

INGREDIENTS

Radix Bupleuri	Chai hu	柴胡
Radix Angelicae Sinensis	Dang gui	當歸
Radix Paeoniae Lactiflorae	Bai shao	白芍
Radix Salviae Miltiorrhizae	Dan shen	丹參
Sclerotium Poriae Cocos	Fu ling	茯苓
Rhizoma Atractylodis Macrocephalae	Bai zhu	白朮
Rhizoma Cyperi Rotundi	Xiang fu	香附
Pericarpium Citri Reticulatae	Chen pi	陳皮
Cortex Moutan Radicis	Mu dan pi	牡丹皮
Fructus Gardeniae Jasminoidis	Zhi zi	梔子
Rhizoma Zingiberis Officinalis	Gan jiang	乾姜
Radix Glycyrrhizae Uralensis	Gan cao	甘草

Xanthium Relieve Surface

INGREDIENTS

Fructus Xanthii Sivirici	Cang er zi	蒼耳子
Flos Chrysanthemi Morifolii	Ju hua	菊花
Radix Astragali Membranacei	Huang qi	黄耆
Radix Ligustici Chuansiong	Chuan xiong	川芎
Herba seu flos Schizonepetae Tenuifoliae	Jing jie	荊芥
CortexPhellodendri	Huang bai	黄柏
Radixx Ledebouriellae Divaricatae	Fang feng	防風
Radix Angelicae Dahuricae	Bai zhi	白芷
Radix Rehmanniae Glutinose Conquitae	Shu di huang	熟地黄
Fructus Pruni Mume	Wu mei	烏梅
Radix Platycodi Grandiflori	Jie geng	桔梗
Herba cum Radice Asari	Xi xin	細辛
Rhizoma Anemarrhenae Aspodeloidis	Zhi mu	知母
Radix Glycyrrhizae Uralensis	Gan cao	甘草

Yin Chao Jin

INGREDIENTS SAME AS YIN QIAO

Yin Chao Junior

INGREDIENTS

Fructus Forsythiae Suspensae	Lian qiao	連翹
Folium Mori Albae	Sang ye	桑葉
Massa Fermentata	Shen qu	神曲
Herba Dendrobii	Shi hu	石斛
Bulbus Fritillariae Thunbergii	Zhe bei mu	浙貝母
Radix Platycodi Grandiflori	Jie geng	桔梗
Folium Eriobotryae Japonicae	Pi pa ye	枇杷葉
Pu er cha	Pu er cha	普洱茶
Microcos pariculata	Po bu ye	破布葉
Pericarpium Trichosanthis	Gua lou pi	瓜蔞皮
Rhizoma Pinelliae Ternatae	Ban xia	半夏

INGREDIENTS CONTINUED FROM PAGE 198

Flos Chrysanthemi Morifolii	Ju hua	菊 花
Herba Menthae Haplocalycis	Bo he	薄 荷
Radix Peucedani	Qian hu	前 胡
Fructus Immaturus Citri Aurantii	Zhi shi	枳 實
Fructus Gardeniae Jasminoidis	Zhi zi	枳 子
Herba Eupatorii Fortunei	Pei lan	佩 蘭
Folium Perillae Frutescentis	Zi su ye	紫 蘇 葉

JADE PHARMACY and K'AN HERBALS

Arouse Vigor

INGREDIENTS

Radix Astragali	Huang qi	黃 耆
Radix Ginseng	Ren shen	人 參
Radix Angelicae Sinensis	Dang gui	當 歸
Radix Glycyrrhizae Uralensis	Zhi gan cao	炙 甘 草
Pericarpium Citri Reticulatae	Chen pi	陳 皮
Rhizoma Cimicifugae	Sheng ma	升 麻
Radix Bupleuri	Chai hu	柴 胡
Rhizoma Atractylodis Macrocephalae	Bai zhu	白 朮

Compassionate Sage

INGREDIENTS

Semen Zizyphi Spinosae	Suan zao ren	酸 棗 仁
Radix Polygalae Tenuifoliae	Yaun zhi	遠 志
Semen Biotae Orientalis	Bai zi ren	柏 子 仁
Succinum	Hu po	琥 珀
Radix Codonopsis Pilosulae	Dang shen	黨 參
Rhizoma Coptidis	Huang lian	黃 連
Rhizoma Acori Graminei	Shi chang pu	石 菖 蒲
Arillus Euphoriae Longanae	Long yan rou	龍 眼 肉

INGREDIENTS CONTINUED FROM PAGE 199

Cortex Albizziae Julibrissin	He huan pi	合 歡 皮
Radix Salviae Miltiorrhizae	Dan shen	丹 參
Os Draconis	Long gu	龍 骨
Radix Angelicae Sinensis	Dang gui	當 歸
Sclerotium Ganodermae	Ling zhi	靈 芝
Sclerotium Poriae Cocos	Fu ling	茯 苓
Radix Glycyrrhizae Uralensis	Gan cao	甘 草

Dispel Invasion

INGREDIENTS SAME AS PRIME RESCUE

Dynamic Warrior

INGREDIENTS

Cortex Eucommiae Ulmoidis	Du zhong	杜 仲
Radix Morindae Officinalis	Ba ji tian	巴 戟 天
Herba Cistanches	Rou cong rong	肉 蓯 蓉
Semen Psoraleae Corylifoliae	Bu gu zhi	補 骨 脂
Cortex Cinnamomi Cassiae	Rou gui	肉 桂
Radix Aconiti Carmichaelai Praeparata	Fu zi	附 子
Frutus Schisandrae Chinensis	Wu wei zi	五 味 子
Achyranthis Bidentatae	Niu xi	牛 膝
Radix Rehmanniae Glutinosae Conquitae	Shu di huang	熟 地 黃
Radix Dioscoreae Oppositae	Shan yao	山 藥
Fructus Corni Officinalis	Shan zhu yu	山 茱 萸
Fructus Lycii Chinensis	Gou qi zi	枸 杞 子
Semen Cuscutae	Tu si zi	兔 絲 子
Radix Angelicae Sinensis	Dang gui	當 歸
Radix Ginseng	Ren shen	人 參

Early Comfort

INGREDIENTS SAME AS PRIME RELIEF

Firm Vessel

INGREDIENTS

Ootheca Mantidis	Sang piao xiao	桑 螵 蛸
Radix Polygale Tenuifoliae	Yuan zhi	遠 志
Rhizoma Acori Graminei	Shi chang pu	石 菖 蒲
Radix Ginseng	Ren shen	人 參
Sclerotium Poriae Cocos	Fu shen	茯 神
Radix Angelicae Sinensis	Dang gui	當 歸
Radix Dioscoreae Oppositae	Shan yao	山 藥
Radix Linderae Strychnifoliae	Wu yao	烏 藥
Fructus Alpiniae Oxyphyllae	Yi zhi ren	益 智 仁
Fructus Schisandrae Chinensis	Wu wei zi	五 味 子
Fructus Corni Officinalis	Shan zhu yu	山 茱 萸
Os Draconis	Long gu	龍 骨

Gather Vitality

INGREDIENTS

Radix Ginseng	Ren shen	人 參
Radix Astragali	Huang qi	黃 耆
Rhizoma Atractylodis Macrocephalae	Bai Zhu	白 朮
Radix Salviae Miltiorrhizae	Dan shen	丹 參
Semen Zizyphi Spinosae	Suan zao ren	酸 棗 仁
Arillus Euphoriae Longanae	Long yan rou	龍 眼 肉
Radix Saussureae seu Vladimiriae	Mu xiang	木 香
Radix Glycyrrhizae Uralensis	Zhi gan cao	炙 甘 草
Radix Angelicae Sinensis	Dang gui	當 歸
Radix Polygale Tenuifoliae Recens	Yuan zhi	遠 志
Rhizoma Zingiberis Officialis Recens	Sheng jiang	生 姜
Fructus Zizyphi Jujubae	Da zao	大 棗

Initial Defense

INGREDIENTS SAME AS PRIME RESPONSE

Lucid Channel

INGREDIENTS SAME AS LUCID CLARITY

Lucid Clarity

INGREDIENTS

Pericarpium Citri Reticulatae	Chen pi	陳 皮
Rhizoma Pinelliae Ternatae	Fa ban xia	法 半 夏
Sclerotium Poriae Cocos	Fu ling	茯 苓
Radix Glycyrrhizae Uralensis	Zhi gan cao	炙 甘 草
Fructus Citri seu Ponciri Immaturus	Zhi si	枳 實
Rhizoma Arisaematis Consanguineum	Tian nan xing	天 南 星
Rhizoma Acori Graminei	Chang pu	菖 蒲

Meridian Circulation

INGREDIENTS

Radix Duhuo	Du huo	獨 活
Radix Gentianae Macrophyllae	Qin jiao	秦 艽
Radix Ledebouriellae Sesloidis	Fang feng	防 風
Ramulus Loranthi seu Visci	Sang ji sheng	桑 寄 生
Cortex Euconmiae Ulmoidis	Du zhong	杜 仲
Radix Cyathulae	Chuan niu xi	川 牛 膝
Cortex Cinnamoni Cassiae	Rou gui	肉 桂
Radix Angelicae Sinensis	Dang gui	當 歸
Radix Paeoniae Lactiflorae	Bai shao	白 芍
Radix Ginseng	Ren shen	人 參
Radix Glycyrrhizae Uralensis	Zhi gan cao	炙 甘 草
Sclerotium Poriae Cocos	Fu ling	茯 苓
Cortex Erythrinae Variegatae	Hai tong pi	海 桐 皮
Radix Aristolochiae seu Cocculi	Guang fang ji	廣 防 己
Rhizoma Cibotii Barometz	Gou ji	狗 脊

Meridian Passage

INGREDIENTS

Flos Carthami Tinctorii	Hong hua	紅 花
Radix Achyranthis Bidentatae	Niu xi	牛 膝
Radix Gentianae Macrophyllae	Qin jiao	秦 艽
Rhizoma et Radix Notopterygii	Qiang huo	羌 活
Radix Ligustici Wallichii	Chuan xiong	川 芎
Radix Angelicae Sinensis	Dang gui	當 歸
Rhizoma Cyperi Rotudi	Xiang fu	香 附
Radix Glycyrrhizae Uralensis	Gan cao	甘 草
Myrrha	Mo yao	沒 藥
Pyritum	Zi ran tong	自 然 銅
Rhizoma Gusuibu	Gu sui bu	骨 碎 補
Radix Paeoniae Lactiflorae	Bai shao	白 芍
Gummi Olibanum	Ru xiang	乳 香

Prime Relief

INGREDIENTS

Herba Angastache seu Pogostemi	Huo xiang	藿 香
Folium Perillae Frutescentis	Su ye	蘇 葉
Pericarpium Citri Reticulatae	Chen pi	陳 皮
Radix Angelicae	Bai zhi	白 芷
Rhizoma Atractylodis Macrocephalae	Bai zhu	白 朮
Cortex Magnoliae Offcinalis	Hou po	厚 樸
Rhizoma Pinelliae Ternatae	Ban xie	半 夏
Sclerotium Poriae Cocos	Fu ling	茯 苓
Radix Saussureae seu Vladimiriae	Mu xiang	木 香

Prime Rescue

INGREDIENTS

Herba seu Flos Schizonepetae Tenuifoliae	Jing jie	荆 芥
Radix Ledebouriellae Sesloidis	Fang feng	防 風
Folium Perillae Frutescentis	Su Ye	蘇 葉
Rhizoma et Radix Notopterygii	Qiang huo	羌 活
Radix Bupleuri	Chai hu	柴 胡
Fructus Citri seu Ponciri	Zhi k	枳 殼
Sclerotium Poriae Cocos	Fu ling	茯 苓
Radix Platycodi Grandiflora	Jie geng	桔 梗
Rhizoma et Radix Ligustici Sinensis	Chuan xiong	川 芎
Radix Glycyrrhizae Uralensis	Zhi gan cao	炙 甘 草
Rhizoma Zingerberis Officinalis Recens	Sheng jiang	生 姜

Prime Response

INGREDIENTS

Flos Lonicerae Japonicae	Yin hua	銀 花
Fructus Forsythiae Suspensae	Lian qiao	連 翹
Folium Mori Albae	Sang ye	桑 葉
Flos Chrysanthemi Morifolii	Ju hua	菊 花
Radix Platycody Grandiflori	Jie geng	桔 梗
Herba Menthae	Bo he	薄 荷
Herba seu Flos Schizonepetae Tenuifoliae	Jing jie	荆 芥
Radix Scorphulariae Ning poensis	Xuan shen	玄 參
Fructus Arctii Lappae	Niu bang zi	牛 蒡 子
Radix Peucedaani	Qian hu	前 胡
Radix Glycyrrhizae Uralensis	Gan cao	甘 草
Rhizoma Zingerberis Officinalis Recens	Sheng jiang	生 姜
Fructus Hordei Vulgaris Germinantus	Mai Ya	麥 芽
Massa Fermentata	Shen qu	神 曲

Prosperous Farmer

INGREDIENTS

Radix Ginseng	Ren shen	人 參
Sclerotium Poriae Cocos	Fu ling	茯 苓
Radix Astragali	Huang qi	黄 耆
Radix Glycyrrhizae Uralensis	Gan cao	甘 草
Radix Dioscoreae Oppositae	Shan yao	山 藥
Rhizoma Zingiberis Officinalis Recens	Sheng jiang	生 姜
Percarpium citri Reticulatae	Chen pi	陳 皮
Rhizoma Pinelliae Ternatae	Ban xia	半 夏
Fructus seu Semen Amomi	Sha ren	砂 仁
Radix Saussureae seu Vladimiriae	Mu xiang	木 香
Cortex Magnoliae Officinalis	Hou po	厚 樸
Fructus Crataegi	Shan zha	山 楂

Quiet Contemplative

INGREDIENTS

Radix Rehmanniae Glutinosae Conquitae	Shu di huang	熟 地 黄
Fructus Corni Officinalis	Shan zhu yu	山 茱 萸
Radix Dioscoreae Oppositae	Shan yao	山 藥
Sclerotium Poriae Cocos	Fu ling	茯 苓
Rhizoma Alismatis Plantago-aquaticae	Ze xie	澤 瀉
Cortex Moutan Radicis	Mu dan pi	牡 丹 皮
Frutus Mori Albae	Sang shen	桑 椹
Frutus Lycii Chinensis	Gou qi zi	枸 杞 子
Radix Polygoni Multiflori	Shou wu	首 烏
Semen Cuscutae	Tu si zi	兔 絲 子
Herba Ecliptae Prostratae	Han lian cao	旱 蓮 草
Frutus Ligustri Lucidi	Nu zhen zi	女 貞 子

Quell Fire

INGREDIENTS

Radix Gentianae Scabrae	Long dan cao	龍 膽 草
Fructus Gardeniae Jasminoidis	Shan zhi zi	山 梔 子
Radix Scutellariae Baicalensis	Huang qin	黃 芩
Radix Bupleuri	Chai hu	柴 胡
Radix Angelicae Sinensis	Dang gui	當 歸
Radix Rehmanniae Glutinosae	Sheng di huang	生 地 黃
Rhizoma Alismatis Plantago-aquaticae	Ze xie	澤 瀉
Semen Plantaginis	Che qian zi	車 前 子
Caulis Mutong	Mu tong	木 通
Radix Glycyrrhizae Uralensis	Gan cao	甘 草

Relaxed Wanderer

INGREDIENTS

Radix Bupleuri	Chai hu	柴 胡
Radix Angelicae Sinensis	Dang gui	當 歸
Cortex Moutan Radicis	Mu dan pi	牡 丹 皮
Rhizoma Atractylodis Macrocephalae	Bai zhu	白 朮
Sclerotium Poriae Cocos	Fu ling	茯 苓
Herba Menthae	Bo he	薄 荷
Redix Glycyrrhizae Uralensis	Gan cao	甘 草
Cortex Moutan Radicis	Mu dan pi	牡 丹 皮
Fructus Gardiniae Jasminoidis	Shan zhi zi	山 梔 子
Radix Ligustici Wallichii	Chuan xiong	川 芎
Rhizoma Gastrodiae Elatae	Tian ma	天 麻
Rhizoma Cyperi Rotundi	Xiang fu	香 附
Rhizoma Zingiberis Officinalis Recens	Sheng jiang	生 姜

Temper Fire

INGREDIENTS

Radix Rhemanniae Glutinosae Conquitae	Shu di huang	熟 地 黄
Fructus Corni Officinalis	Shan zhu yu	山 茱 萸
Radix Dioscoreae Oppositae	Shan yao	山 藥
Rhizoma Alismatis Plantago-aquaticae	Ze xie	澤 瀉
Cortex Moutan Radicis	Mu dan pi	牡 丹 皮
Sclerotium Poriae Cocos	Fu ling	茯 苓
Radix Amenmarrhenae	Zhi mu	知 母
Cortex Phellodendri	Huang bai	黄 柏

Wise Judge

INGREDIENTS

Radix Glehniae Littoralis	Sha Shen	沙 參
Tuber Ophiopogonis Japonici	Mai men dong	麥 門 冬
Rhizoma Polygonati Odorati	Yu zhu	玉 竹
Tuber Asparagi Cochinchinensis	Tian men dong	天 門 冬
Bulbus Lilii	Bai he	百 合
Radix Platycodi Grandiflori	Jie geng	桔 梗
Bulbus Fritillariae Thunbergii	Zhe bei mu	浙 貝 母
Radix Angelicae Sinensis	Dang gui	當 歸
Radix Rehmanniae Glutinosae Conquite	Shu di huang	熟 地 黄
Fructificatio tremellae Fuciformis	Bai mu er	白 木 耳
Radix Panacis Quinquefolii	Xi yang shen	西 洋 參
Radix Glycyrrhizae Uralensis	Gan cao	甘 草
Sclerotium Poriae Cocos	Fu ling	茯 苓
Radix Pseudostellariae Heterophyllae	Tai zi shen	太 子 參
Fructus Schisandrae Chinensis	Wu wei zi	五 味 子

Women's Journey

INGREDIENTS		
Fructus Evodiae	Wu zhu yu	吳 茱 萸
Radix Angelicae Sinensis	Dang gui	當 歸
Radix Paeoniae Lactiflorae	Bai shao	白 芍
Radix Ginseng	Ren shen	人 參
Ramulus Cinnamomi	Gui zhi	桂 枝
Gelatinum Asini	E jiao	阿 膠
Cortex Moutan	Mu dan pi	牡 丹 皮
Rhizoma Zingiberis	Sheng jiang	生 姜
Radix Glycyrrhizae	Gan cao	甘 草
Tuber Ophiopogonis	Mai dong	麥 冬
Radix Anemarrhenae	Zhi mu	知 母
Cortex Phellodendri	Huang bai	黃 柏
Radix Rehmanniae	Sheng di huang	生 地 黃
Rhizoma Curculiginis	Xian mao	仙 茅
Concha Ostreae	Mu li	牡 蠣

Women's Chamber

INGREDIENTS SAME AS WOMEN'S PALACE

Women's Palace

INGREDIENTS		
Ramulus Cinnamomi	Gui zhi	桂 枝
Sclerotium Poriae Cocos	Fu ling	茯 苓
Cortex Moutan	Mu dan pi	牡 丹 皮
Semen Persicae	Tao ren	桃 仁
Radix Paeoniae	Chi shao	赤 芍
Rhizoma Sparganii	San leng	三 稜
Rhizoma Curcumae zedoariae	E zhu	莪 朮
Radix Achyranthis	Niu xi	牛 膝
Rhizoma Cyperi	Xiang fu	香 附
Rhizoma Corydalis	Yan hu suo	延 胡 索
Radix Salviae	Dan shen	丹 參
Radix Glycyrrhizae	Gan cao	甘 草

Women's Precious

INGREDIENTS

Radix Angelica Sinensis	Dang gui	當 歸
Radix Paeoniae Lactiflorae	Bai shao	白 芍
Radix Rehmanniae Glutinosae Conquitae	Shu di huang	熟 地 黃
Radix Ligustici Wallichii	Chuan xiong	川 芎
Radix Ginseng	Ren shen	人 參
Rhizoma Atractylodis Macrocephale	Bai zhu	白 朮
Sclerotium Poriae Cocos	Fu ling	茯 苓
Radix Glycyrrhizae Uralensis	Zhi gan cao	炙 甘 草
Herba Leonuri Heterophylli	Yi mu cao	益 母 草
Radix Polygoni Multiflori	Shou wu	首 烏
Fructus Lycii Chinensis	Gou qi zi	枸 杞 子

Women's Rhythm

INGREDIENTS

Radix Angelica Sinensis	Dang gui	當 歸
Rhizoma Cyperi Rotundi	Xiang fu	香 附
Flos Carthami Tinctorii	Hong hua	紅 花
Pericarpium Citri Reticulatae Viride	Qing pi	青 皮
Rhizoma Alismatis Plantego-aquaticae	Ze xie	澤 瀉
Radix Saussureae seu Vladimiriae	Mu xiang	木 香
Fructus C rataegi	Shan zha	山 楂
Rhizoma Corydalis Yanhusua	Yan hu suo	延 胡 索
Radix Achyranthis Bidentatae	Niu xi	牛 膝
Cortex Cinnamoni Cassiae	Rou gui	肉 桂
Cortex Moutan Radicis	Mu dan pi	牡 丹 皮
Radix Paeoniae Lactiflorae	Bai shao	白 芍
Radix Ligustici Wallichii	Chuan xiong	川 芎
Radix Rehmanniae Glutinosae Conquitae	Shu di huang	熟 地 黃
Cortex Albizziae Julibrissin	He huan pi	合 歡 皮

TURTLE MOUNTAIN

Green Tiger

INGREDIENTS

Fructus Lycii	Gou qi zi	枸 杞 子
Rhizoma Gastrodiae	Tian ma	天 麻
Radix Paeoniae	Bai shao	白 芍
Ramulus Uncariae	Gou teng	鉤 藤
Fructus Pruni Mume	Wu mei	烏 梅
Fructusa Corni	Shan zhu yu	山 茱 萸
Cortex Eucomiae	Du zhong	杜 仲
Radix Rehmanniae	Sheng di huang	生 地 黃
Fructus Meliae Toosendan	Chuan lian zi	川 楝 子
Rhizoma Corydalis	Yan hu suo	延 胡 索
Radix Ligustici	Chuan xiong	川 芎
Cortex Moutan	Mu dan pi	牡 丹 皮
Flos Chrysanthemi	Ju hua	菊 花
Radix Bupleuri	Chai hu	柴 胡
Radix Polygoni Multiflori	He shou wu	何 首 烏
Rhizoma Alismatis	Ze xie	澤 瀉
Radix Angelicae Sinensis	Dang gui	當 歸
Fructus Gardeniae	Zhi zi	梔 子
Rhizoma Coptidis	Huang lian	黃 連
Cormu Antelopis	Ling yang jiao	羚 羊 角

Lower Burner

INGREDIENTS

Semen Plantaginis	Che qian zi	車 前 子
Herba Dianthi	Qu mai	瞿 麥
Herba Polygoni Avicularis	Bian xu	萹 蓄
Talcum Hua shi	Hua shi	滑 石
Fructus Gardinia	Zhi zi	梔 子
Caulis Mutong	Mu tong	木 通
Radix Glycyrrhizae	Gan cao	甘 草

Medulla Junci	Deng xin cao	燈芯草
Cornu Cervi Parvum	Lu rong	鹿茸
Adrenal Gland	Shen shang xian	腎上腺
Cordyceps	Dong chong xia cao	冬蟲夏草
Fructus Cnidii	She chuang zi	蛇床子
Rhizoma Smilacis	Tu fu ling	土茯苓
Rhizoma Curculiginis	Xian mao	仙茅
Herba Epimedii	Yin yang huo	淫羊藿
Smithsonite	Lu gan shi	爐甘石
Herba Lysimachiae	Jin qian cao	金錢草
Cortex Phellodendri	Huang bai	黄柏

Middle Burner

INGREDIENTS

Radix Ginseng	Ren shen	人參
Sclerotium Poriae Cocos	Fu ling	茯苓
Rhizoma Atractylodis	Bai zhu	白朮
Radix Glycyrrhizae	Gan cao	甘草
Semen Nelumbins	Lian zi	蓮子
Semen Coicis	Yi yi ren	薏苡仁
Semen Dolichoris	Bai bian dou	白扁豆
Rhizoma Dioscorea	Shan yao	山藥
Fructus Amomi	Sha ren	砂仁
Radix Platycodi	Jie geng	桔梗
Calculus Bovis	Niu huang	牛黄
Pancreas Gland	Yi xian	胰腺
Fructus Chaenomelis	Mu gua	木瓜
Fructus Psoreleae	Bu gu zi	補骨脂
Flos Magnoliae liliflor	Xin yi hua	辛荑花
Radix Pulsatillae	Bai tou weng	白頭翁
Cortex Ailanthus	Chun gen pi	椿根皮
Rhizoma Coptidis	Huang lian	黄連

Red Horse

INGREDIENTS

Radix Panas Ginseng	Ren shen	人 參
Fructus Schisandra	Wu wei zi	五 味 子
Radix Saussureae	Mu xiang	木 香
Rhizoma Coptidis	Huang lian	黃 連
Rhizoma Acori Graminei	Chang pu	菖 蒲
Radix Peaoniae Rubra	Chi shao	赤 芍
Radix Salviae	Dan shen	丹 參
Radix Polygalae	Yuan zhi	遠 志
Radix Pseudoginseng	San qi	三 七
Sclerotium Poriae Cocos	Fu ling	茯 苓
Tuber Ophiopogonis	Mai men dong	麥 門 冬
Margarita	Zhen zhu	珍 珠
Calcined Magnetite	Ci shi	磁 石
Fructus Longanae	Long yan rou	龍 眼 肉
Ganodermae Lucidum	Ling zhi	靈 芝
Radix Glycyrhizae	Gan cao	甘 草
Semen Ziziphi	Suan zao ren	酸 棗 仁
Fructus Leonturi	Chong wei zi	茺 蔚 子
Os Draconis	Long gu	龍 骨
Cortex Albizziae	He huang pi	合 歡 皮
Cortex Cinnamomi	Gui zhi	桂 枝
Semen Biotae	Bai zi	白 芷
Succinum	Hu po	琥 珀

Upper Burner

INGREDIENTS SAME AS PRIME RELIFE

White Turtle

INGREDIENTS

Semen Seami	Hei zhi ma	黑 芝 麻
Radix Rehmannai	Di huang	地 黃
Fructus Lycii	Gou qi zi	枸 杞 子

INGREDIENTS CONTINUED FROM PAGE 212

Herba Eclipta	Han lian cao	旱蓮草
Fructus Rosae	Jin ying zi	金櫻子
Fructus Ligustri	Nu zhen zi	女貞子
Rhizoma Polygonati	Huang jing	黃精
Semen Cuscuta	Tu si zi	兔絲子
Morus alba	Sang shen	桑椹
Semen Euryales	Qian shi	芡實
Radix Achyranthes	Niu xi	牛膝
Fructus Cornus	Shan zhu yu	山茱萸
Radix Dioscoreae	Shan yao	山藥
Sclerotium Poriae Cocos	Fu ling	茯苓
Cortes Phellodendron	Huang bai	黃柏
Fructus Schisandra	Wu wei zi	五味子
Rhiaoma Alisma	Ze xia	澤夏
Cortex Moutan	Mu dan pi	牡丹皮
Rhizoma Anemarrhena	Zhi mu	知母
Royal jelly	Feng ru	峰乳

K'AN HERBALS (Traditionals)

Akebia Relieving Formula

INGREDIENTS

Caulis Mutong	Mu tong	木通
Herba Dianthi	Qu mai	瞿麥
Herba Polygoni Avicularis	Bian xu	萹蓄
Medulla Junci	Deng xin cao	燈芯草
Talcum	Hua shi	滑石
Semen Plantaginis	Che qian zi	車前子
Fructus Gardiniae Jasminoidis	Shan zhi zi	山梔子
Radix et Rhizoma Rhei	Da huang	大黃
Radix Glycyrrhizae Uralensis	Gan cao	甘草

Bi Yan Plan

INGREDIENTS

Fructus Xanthii Sivirici	Cang er zi	蒼耳子
Flos Magnoliae liliflor	Xin yi hua	辛荑花
Radix Glycyrrhizae Uralensis	Gan cao	甘草
Cortex Phellodendri	Huang bai	黃柏
Radix Platycodi Grandiflori	Jie geng	桔梗
Frutus Schisandrae Chinensis	Wu wei zi	五味子
Fructus Forsythiae Suspensae	Lian qiao	連翹
Radix Angelicae	Bai zhi	白芷
Radix Anemarrhenae	Zhi mu	知母
Flos Chrysanthemi Indici	Ye ju hua	野菊花
Radix Ledebouriellae Sesloidis	Fang feng	防風
Herba seu Flos Schizonepetae Tenuifoliae	Jing jie	荆芥

Calm Dragon Formula

INGREDIENTS

Radix Bupleuri	Chai hu	柴胡
Radix Scutellariae Baicalensis	Huang qin	黃芩
Rhizoma Pinelliae Ternatae	Ban xia	半夏
Radix Ginseng	Ren shen	人參
Concha Ostreae	Mu li	牡蠣
Os Draconis	Long gu	龍骨
Ramulus Cinnamomi	Gui zhi	桂枝
Sclerotium Poriae Cocos	Fu ling	茯苓
Fructus Zizyphi Jujubae	Da zao	大棗
Rhizoma Zingiberis Officinalis	Gan jiang	乾姜
Haematitum	Dai zhe shi	代赭石
Fructus Gardiniae Jasminoidis	Shan zhi zi	山梔子

Celestial Emperor's Blend

INGREDIENTS

Radix Rehmanniae Gluti8nosae	Sheng di huang	生 地 黄
Radix Scrophulariae Ningpoensis	Xuan shen	玄 參
Fructus Schisandrae Chinensis	Wu wei zi	五 味 子
Radix Aspariagi Cochinchinensis	Tian men dong	天 門 冬
Radix Ophinopogonis Japonici	Mai men dong	麥 門 冬
Radix Angelicae Sinensis	Dang gui	當 歸
Semen Biotae Orientalis	Bai zi ren	柏 子 仁
Semen Zizyphi Jujubae	Suan zao ren	酸 棗 仁
Radix Polygalae Tenuifoliae	Yuan zhi	遠 志
Sclerotium Poriae Cocos	Fu ling	茯 苓
Radix Salviae Miltiorrhizae	Dan shen	丹 參
Radix Codonopsis Pilosulae	Dang shen	黨 參
Radix Platycodi Grandiflori	Jie geng	桔 梗

Colorful Phoenix Pearl Combo

INGREDIENTS

Margarita	Zhen Zhu	珍 珠
Concha Margaritifera	Zhen zhu mu	珍 珠 母
Radix Rehmanniae Glutinosae Conquita	Shu di huang	熟 地 黄
Radix Adenophorae Tetraphylla	Nan sha shen	南 沙 參
Radix Scrophulariae Ningpoensis	Xuan shen	玄 參
Cortex Phellodendri	Huang bai	黄 柏
Radix et Rhizoma Rhei	Sheng di huang	生 地 黄
Cornu Saigae Tataricae	Ling yang jiao	羚 羊 角

Copticlear

INGREDIENTS

Rhizoma Coptidis	Huang lian	黄 連

Copticetox

INGREDIENTS

Rhizoma Coptidis	Huang lian	黄 連
Radix Scutellariae Baicalensis	Huang qin	黄 芩
Cortex Phellodendri	Huang bai	黄 柏
Fructus Gardiniae Jasminoidis	Shan zhi zi	山 梔 子

Free and Easy Wanderer

INGREDIENTS

Radix Bupleuri	Chai hu	柴 胡
Radix Paeoniae Lactiflorae	Bai shao	白 芍
Radix Angelicae Sinensis	Dang gui	當 歸
Sclerotium Poriae Cocos	Fu ling	茯 苓
Rhizoma Atractylodis Macrocephalae	Bai zhu	白 朮
Rhizoma Zingiberis Officinalis	Gan jiang	乾 姜
Herba Menthae	Bo he	薄 荷
Radix Glycyrrhizae Uralensis	Gan cao	甘 草

Gan Mao Ling

INGREDIENTS

Ilex Pubescens Hook. Et Arn	Mao dong qing	毛 冬 青
Fructus Evodiae	Wu zhu yu	吳 茱 萸
Radix Isatidis seu Baphicacanthi	Ban lan gen	板 蘭 根
Flos Chrysanthemi Morifolii	Huang ju hua	黄 菊 花
Flos Lonicerae Japonicae	Jin yin hua	金 銀 花

Hemmorease

INGREDIENTS

Radix Pseudoginseng	San qi	三 七
Fructus Sophorae Japonica	Huai jiao	槐 角
Folium Callicarpae	Zi zhu cao	紫 珠 草
Radix Ledebouriellae Sesloidis	Fang feng	防 風
Rhizoma Atractylodis Macrocephalae	Bai zhu	白 朮
Radix Scutellariae Baicalensis	Huang qin	黃 芩
Fructus Citri Aurantii	Zhi ke	枳 殼
Fructus Gardiniae Jasminoidis	Shan zhi zi	山 梔 子
Calla Rhoia Chinensis	Wu bei zi	五 倍 子
Radix Sanguisorbae Officinalis	Di yu	地 榆

Invigorate the Collaterals

INGREDIENTS

Radix Angelicae Sinensis	Dang gui	當 歸
Radix Salviae Miltiorrhizae	Dan shen	丹 參
Gummi Olibanum	Ru xiang	乳 香
Myrrha	Mo yao	沒 藥
Rhizoma Corydalis	Yan hu suo	延 胡 索
Radix Achyranthis Bidentatae	Niu xi	牛 膝

Jade Windscreen

INGREDIENTS

Radix Astragali	Huang qi	黃 耆
Rhizoma Atractylodis Macrocephalae	Bai zhu	白 朮
Radix Ledebouriellae Sesloidis	Fang feng	防 風
Radix Dioscoreae Oppositae	Shan yao	山 藥
Fructus Zizyphi Jujubae	Hei zao	黑 棗
Ramulus Cinnamomi	Gui zhi	桂 枝
Radix Paeoniae Lactiflorae	Bai shao	白 芍

Li Dan Support

INGREDIENTS

Radix Scutellariae Baicalensis	Huang qin	黄芩
Radix Saussureae seu Vladimiriae	Mu xiang	木香
Herba Lysimachiae	Jin qian cao	金錢草
Flos Lonicerae Japonicae	Jin yin hua	金銀花
Radix Bupleuri	Chai hu	柴胡
Folium Daqingye	Da qing ye	大青葉
Herba Artemisiae Yinchenhao	Yin chen	茵陳
Radix et Rhizoma Rhei	Da huang	大黄

Minor Bupleurum

INGREDIENTS

Radix Bupleuri	Chai hu	柴胡
Radix Scutellariae Baicalensis	Huang qin	黄芩
Rhizoma Pinelliae Ternatae	Ban xia	半夏
Radix Ginseng	Ren shen	人參
Radix Glycyrrhizae Uralensis	Zhi gan cao	炙甘草
Fructus Zizyphi Jujubae	Hong zao	紅棗
Rhizoma Zingiberis Officinalis Recens	Sheng jiang	生姜

Pinellia Phlegm Dispersing Formula

INGREDIENTS

Rhizoma Pinelliae Ternatae	Ban xia	半夏
Rhizoma Arisaematis Consanguineum	Tian nan xing	天南星
Semen Trichosanthis Kirilowii	Gua lou ren	瓜蔞仁
Fructus Immaturus Citri Aurantii	Zhi shi	枳實
Pars Rubra Epicarpii Citri Erythrocarpae	Ju hong	桔紅
Semen Pruni Armeniacae	Ku xing ren	苦杏仁
Sclerotium Poriae Cocos	Fu ling	茯苓

Smooth Response

INGREDIENTS

Radix et Rhizoma Rhei	Sheng di huang	生 地 黄
Extremitas Radicis Angelicae Sinensis	Dang gui wei	當 歸 尾
Rhizoma Et Radix Notopterygii	Qiang huo	羌 活
Semen Persicae	Tao ren	桃 仁
Semen Cannabis Satvae	Huo ma ren	火 麻 仁

Water's Way

INGREDIENTS

Rhizoma Alismatis Orientalis	Ze xia	澤 瀉
Sclertium Poriae Cocos	Fu ling	茯 苓
Sclerotium Polypori Umbellati	Zhu ling	豬 苓
Radix Stephaniae Tetrandrae	Han fang ji	漢 防 己
Rhizoma Atractyloidis	Cang zhu	蒼 朮
Rhizoma Atractyylodis Macrocephalae	Bai zhu	白 朮
Ramulus Cinnamomi Cassiae	Gui zhi	桂 枝

Yin Qiao

INGREDIENTS

Flos Lonicerae Japonicae	Jin yin hua	金 銀 花
Fructus Forsythiae Suspensae	Lian qiao	連 翹
Radix Platycodi Grandiflori	Jie geng	桔 梗
Fructus Arctii Lappae	Niu bang zi	牛 蒡 子
Herba Menthae Haplocalycis	Bo he	薄 荷
Semen Sojae Praeparatum	Dan dou chi	淡 豆 豉
Herba seu Flos Schizenepetae Tenuifolia	Jing jie	荆 芥
Herba Lophatheri Gracilis	Dan zhu ye	淡 竹 葉
Rhizoma Phragmitis Communis	Lu gen	蘆 根
Radix Glycyrrhizae Uralinsis	Gan cao	甘 草

LONG LIFE HERBAL PHARMACY

Allergease

INGREDIENTS

Herba cum Raice Asari	Xi xin	細 辛
Ramulus Cinnamomi	Gui zhi	桂 枝
Radix Glycyrrhizae Uralensis	Gan cao	甘 草
Radix Scutellariae Baicalensis	Huang qin	黃 芩
Herba Ephedrae	Ma huang	麻 黃
Radix Astragali	Huang qi	黃 耆
Radix Ledebouriellae Sesloidis	Fang feng	防 風
Rhizoma Atractylodis Macrocephalae	Bai zhu	白 朮

Five Detox

INGREDIENTS

Flos Lonicerae Japonicae	Jin yin hua	金 銀 花
Flos Chrysanthemi Indici	Ye ju hua	野 菊 花
Herba Taraxaci Mongolici cum Radice	Pu gong ying	蒲 公 英
Herba cum Radice Violae Yedoensitis	Zi hua di ding	紫 花 地 丁
Radix Semiaquilegia	Zi bei tian kui	紫 背 天 葵

Herpecream

INGREDIENTS

Herba Aloes	Lu hui	蘆 薈
Rhizoma Pleione	Shan ci gu	山 慈 菇
Calla Rhoia Chinensis	Wu bei zi	五 倍 子
Radix Lithospermi seu Arnebiae	Zi cao	紫 草
Gypsum Shi gao	Shi gao	石 膏
Vitamin E		

Liver Pacifier

INGREDIENTS

Radix Paeoniae Lactiflorae	Bai shao	白 芍
Radix Glycyrrhizae Uralensis	Gan cao	甘 草
Fructus Citri Aurantii	Zhi ke	枳 殼
Radix Ligustici Wallichii	Chuan xiong	川 芎
Rhizoma Cyperi Rotudi	Xiang fu	香 附
Pericarpium Citri Reticulatae Viride	Qing pi	青 皮
Pericarpium Citri Reticulatae	Chen pi	陳 皮
Tuber Curcumae	Yu jin	郁 金

Si Miao San

INGREDIENTS

Cortex Phellodendri	Huang bai	黄 柏
Rhizoma Atractyloidis	Cang zhu	蒼 朮
Radix Achyranthis Bidentatae	Niu xi	牛 膝
Semen Coicis	Yi yi ren	薏 苡 仁

Skin Cleanser

INGREDIENTS

Radix Astragali	Huang qi	黄 耆
Flos Lonicerae Japonicae	Jin yin hua	金 銀 花
Rhizoma Atractyloidis	Cang zhu	蒼 朮
Radix Rehmanniae Glutinosae	Sheng di huang	生 地 黄
Cortex Moutan Radicis	Mu dan pi	牡 丹 皮
Radix Paeoniae	Chi shao	赤 芍
Radix Sophorae Flavescentis	Ku shen	苦 參
Cortex Dictamni Radicis	Bai xian pi	白 蘚 皮
Cortex Phellodendri	Huang bai	黄 柏
Agkistrodon	Qi she	祈 蛇
Periostracum Cicadae	Chan tui	蟬 蜕
Radix et Rhizoma Rhei	Da huang	大 黄

Uteus A

INGREDIENTS

Radix Angelicae Sinensis	Dang gui	當 歸
Radix Ligustici Wallichii	Chuan xiong	川 芎
Semen Persicae	Tao ren	桃 仁
Rhizoma Zingiberis Officialis Recens prepared	Pao jiang	炮 姜
Radix Glycyrrhizae Uralensis	Zhi gan cao	炙 甘 草
Herba Leonuri Heterophylli	Yi mu cao	益 母 草

Xiao Yao Wan Plus

INGREDIENTS

Cortex Moutan Radicis	Mu dan pi	牡 丹 皮
Fructus Gardeniae Jasminoidis	Shan zhi zi	山 梔 子
Radix Bupleuri	Chai hu	柴 胡
Radix Angelicae Sinensis	Dang gui	當 歸
Sclerotium Poriae Cocos	Fu ling	茯 苓
Radix Paeoniae Lactiflorae	Bai shao	白 芍
Radix Glycyrrhizae Uralensis	Gan cao	甘 草
Rhizoma Atractylodis Macrocephalae	Bai zhu	白 术
Rhizoma Zingiberis Officialis Recens	Sheng jiang	生 姜
Herba Menthae	Bo he	薄 荷

METAGENICS

TCM 2

INGREDIENTS		
Semen Coicis	Yi yi ren	薏苡仁
Radix Stephaniae Tetrandrae	Han fang ji	漢防己
Pericarpium Zanthoxyli Bungeani	Chuan jiao	川椒
Rhizoma Atractyloidis	Cang zhu	蒼朮
Radix Achyranthis Bidentatae	Niu xi	牛膝
Ramulus Cinnamomi	Gui zhi	桂枝
Radix Gentianae Macrophyllae	Qin jiao	秦艽
Radix Duhuo	Du huo	獨活
Herba Ephedrae	Ma huang	麻黃
Rhizoma Zingiberis Officialis Recens	Sheng jiang	生姜
Radix Aconiti Carmichaelai Praeparata	Fu zi	附子
Aconitum Kusnezoffii	Wu tou	烏頭

TCM 4

INGREDIENTS		
Radix Dipsaci Asperi	Xu duan	續斷
Cortex Eucommiae Ulmoidis	Du zhong	杜仲
Rhizoma Polygonati	Huang jing	黃精
Rhizoma Gusuibu	Gu sui bu	骨碎補
Rhizoma Cibotii Barometz	Gou ji	狗脊
Frutus Ligustri Lucidi	Nu zhen zi	女貞子
Radix Glycyrrhizae Uralensis	Gan cao	甘草
Gecko	Ge jie	蛤蚧
Radix Angelicae Sinensis	Dang gui	當歸
Radix Codonopsis Pilosulae	Dang shen	黨參
Radix Astragali	Huang qi	黃耆
Sclerotium Poriae Cocos	Fu ling	茯苓
Radix Dioscoreae Oppositae	Shan yao	山藥
Fructus Chaenomelis	Mu gua	木瓜
Radix Morindae Officinalis	Ba ji tian	巴戟天
Rhizoma Atractylodis Macrocephalae	Bai zhu	白朮

TCM 7

INGREDIENTS

Radix Rehmanniae Glutinosae Conquitae	Shu di huang	熟 地 黄
Radix Dioscoreae Oppositae	Shan yao	山 藥
Fructus Corni Officinalis	Shan zhu yu	山 茱 萸
Cortex Moutan Radicis	Mu dan pi	牡 丹 皮
Sclerotium Poriae Cocos	Fu ling	茯 苓
Rhizoma Alismatis Plantago-aquaticae	Ze xie	澤 瀉

TCM 14

INGREDIENTS

Radix Codonopsis Pilosulae	Dang shen	黨 參
Radix Trichosanthis Kirilowii	Tian hua fen	天 花 粉
Radix Puerariae	Ge gen	葛 根
Tuber Ophiopogonis Japonici	Mai men dong	麥 門 冬
Sclerotium Poriae Cocos	Fu ling	茯 苓
Radix Rehmanniae Glutinosae	Sheng di huang	生 地 黄
Radix Astragali	Huang qi	黄 耆
Fructus Pruni Mume	Wu mei	烏 梅
Frutus Schisandrae Chinensis	Wu wei zi	五 味 子
Radix Glycyrrhizae Uralensis	Gan cao	甘 草

PACIFIC BIOLOGIC

APF-7

INGREDIENTS

Frutus Schisandrae Chinensis	Wu wei zi	五 味 子
Folium Ginkgo Bilobae	Bai guo ye	白 果 葉
Radix Astragali	Huang qi	黃 耆
Pericarpium Citri Reticulatae	Chen pi	陳 皮
Radix Paeoniae Lactiflorae	Bai shao	白 芍
Radix Glycyrrhizae Uralensis	Gan cao	甘 草
Herba Epimedii	Yin yang huo	淫 羊 藿
Siberian ginseng		
Cordyseps		

PRO BOTANIXX

Arthritis

INGREDIENTS

Radix Bupleuri	Chai hu	柴 胡
Radix Scutellariae	Huang qin	黃 芩
Flos Magnliae	Xin yi	辛 夷
Radix Angekicae Dauricae	Bai zhi	白 芷
Rhizoma Cimicifugae	Sheng ma	升 麻
Rhizoma Ligustici	Chuan xiong	川 芎
Herba Asari	Xi xin	細 辛
Rhizoma Notopterygii	Qiang huo	羌 活
Radix Ledebouriellae	Fang feng	防 風
Caulis Akebiae	Mu tong	木 通
Tuber Pinelliae	Ban xia	半 夏
Radix Ginseng	Ren shen	人 參
Radix Glycerrhizae	Gan cao	甘 草
Rhizoma Zingiberis	Sheng jiang	生 姜
Fructus Zizyphi	Da zao	大 棗
Folium Cammellia	Cha Ye	茶 葉

Arthritis (AR-125)

INGREDIENTS

Rhizoma Notopterygii	Qiang huo	羌 活
Radix Angelicae Tuhuo	Du huo	獨 活
Radix Clematadis	Wei ling xian	威 靈 仙
Herba Pycnostelmae	Xu chang qing	徐 長 卿
Radix Achyranthis	Niu xi	牛 膝
Caulis Mucunae	Ji xue teng	雞 血 藤
Gummi Olibanum	Ru xiang	乳 香
Myrrha Mo yao	®S √*f*	沒 藥
Radix Corydalis Yanhusuo	Yan hu suo	延 胡 索
Herba cum Radix Asari	Xi xin	細 辛
Ramulus Cinnamomi	Gui zhi	桂 枝

Arthritis with Weak Constitution (AR-127)

INGREDIENTS

Radix Astragali	Huang qi	黃 耆
Radix Gianseng	Ren shen	人 參
Rhizoma Atractylodos	Bai zhu	白 朮
Radix Glecrrhizae	Gan cao	甘 草
Radix Angelicae	Dang gui	當 歸
Radix Rehmanniae	Di huang	地 黃
Radix Paeoniae	Shao yao	芍 藥
Rhizoma Ligustici	Chuan xiong	川 芎
Cortex Eucommiae	Du zhong	杜 仲
Radix Achyranthis	Niu xi	牛 膝
Gummi Olibanum	Ru xiang	乳 香
Rhizoma Notopterygii	Qiang huo	羌 活
Radix Clematidis	Wei ling xian	威 靈 仙
Radix Ledebouriellae	Fang feng	防 風
Fructus Zizphi	Da Zao	大 棗
Rhizoma Zingiberis	Sheng jiang	生 姜

Asthma (AS-137)

INGREDIENTS

Herba Ephedrae	Ma haung	麻 黄
Semen Ginko	Yin xing	銀 杏
Semen Armeniacae	Xing ren	杏 仁
Semen Perillae	Zi su zi	紫 蘇 子
Tuber Pinelliae	Ban xia	半 夏
Flos Tassilaginis	Kuan dong hua	款 冬 花
Cortex Mori Radicis	Sang bai pi	桑 白 皮
Padix Scutellariae	Huang qin	黄 芩
Radix Glycyrrhizae	Gan cao	甘 草

Blood Circulation (BC-147)

INGREDIENTS

Semen Persicae	Tao ren	桃 仁
Flos Carthami	Hong hua	紅 花
Radix Angelicae	Dang gui	當 歸
Rhizoma Ligustici	Chuan xiong	川 芎
Radix Paoeniae Rubra	Chi shao	赤 芍
Radix Rehmanniae	Di huang	地 黄
Ramulus Cinnamomi	Gui zhi	桂 枝
Radix Bupleuri	Chai hu	柴 胡
Fructus Aurantii	Zhi ke	枳 殼
Radix Glycyrrhizae	Gan cao	甘 草
Radix Achyranthis	Niu xi	牛 膝
Radix Platycodi	Jie geng	桔 梗

Blood Sugar Metabolism Tonic (GL-325)

INGREDIENTS

Radix Ginseng	Ren shen	人 參
Radix Astragali	Huang qi	黄 耆
Rhizoma Atractylodis	Bai zhu	白 朮
Poria	Fu ling	茯 苓

INGREDIENTS CONTINUED FROM PAGE 227

Radix Glycyrrhizae	Gan cao	甘 草
Saccharum Granorum	Jiao tang	膠 糖
Radix Angelicae	Dang gui	當 歸
Radix Rehmannia	Di huang	地 黃
Rhizoma Ligustici	Chuan xiong	川 芎
Radix Paeoniae	Shao yao	芍 藥
Ramulus Cinnamomi	Gui zhi	桂 枝
Fructus Zizyphi	Da zao	大 棗
Rhizoma Zingiberis	Sheng jiang	生 姜

Cardiovascular Disease (VA-841)

INGREDIENTS

Radix Salviae Miltiorrhizae	Dan shen	丹 參
Radix Paeoniae Rubra	Chi shao	赤 芍
Rhizoma Ligustici	Chuan xiong	川 芎
Flos Carthami Tinctorii	Hong hua	紅 花
Dalbergia Odorifera	Jiang xiang	降 香

Candidiasos/Cystitis (CY-207)

INGREDIENTS

Radix Gentiana Scabrae	Long dan cao	龍 膽 草
Cortex Dictamni Radicis	Bai xian pi	白 蘚 皮
Radix Sophorae	Ku shen	苦 參
Fructus Kochiae	Di fu zi	地 膚 皮
Radix Scutellariae	Huang qin	黃 芩
Fructus Gardeniae	Zhi zi	枳 子
Rhizoma Alismatis	Ze xie	澤 瀉
Caulis Akebiae	Mu tong	木 通
Semen Plantaginis	Che qian zi	車 前 子
Radix Angelicae	Dang gui	當 歸
Radix Rehmanniae	Sheng di huang	生 地 黃
Radix Bupleuri	Chai hu	柴 胡
Radix Glycyrrhizae	Gan cao	甘 草

Common Cold Conformation (CO-195)

INGREDIENTS		
Herba Ephedrae	Ma huang	麻 黄
Folium Perillae	Zi su ye	紫 蘇 葉
Bulbus Allii Fistulosi	Cong bai	蔥 白
Rhiaoma Zingiberis	Sheng jiang	生 姜
Radis Angelicae Dahuricae	Bai zhi	白 芷
Radix Puerariae	Ge gen	葛 根
Rhizoma Cimicifugae	Sheng ma	升 麻
Exocarpium Citri Leiocapae	Chen pi	陳 皮
Rhizoma Cyperi	Xiang fu	香 附
Rhizoma Ligustici	Chuan xiong	川 芎

Cold and Flu Heat Conformation (CO-197)

INGREDIENTS		
Flos Lonicerae	Jin yin hua	金 銀 花
Fructus Forsythiae	Lian qiao	連 翹
Radix Platycodi	Jie geng	桔 梗
Fructus Arctii	Niu bang zi	牛 蒡 子
Herba Mentae	Bo he	薄 荷
Herba Schizonepetae	Jing jie	荆 芥
Rhizoma Phragmitis	Lu gen	蘆 根
Folium Bambusae	Zhu ru	竹 茹
Radix Glycyrrhizae	Gan cao	甘 草

Cholesterol Reduction (CR-201)

INGREDIENTS		
Fructus Crataegi	Shan zha	山 楂
Flos Chrysanthemi	Ju hua	菊 花
Radix Polygoni Multiflori	He shou wu	何 首 烏
Semen Cassia Tarae	Jue ming zi	決 明 子
Folium Nelumbinis	He ye	荷 葉
Rhizoma Alismatis	Ze xie	澤 瀉
Rhizoma Polygoni Cuspidati	Hu zhang	虎 杖
Rhizoma Rhei	Da huang	大 黃

Diuretic (DI-221)

INGREDIENTS

Rhizoma Alismatis	Ze xie	澤 瀉
Polyporus	Zhu ling	豬 苓
Poria	Fu ling	茯 苓
Semen Plantaganis	Che qian zi	車 前 子
Rhizoma Atractylodis	Bai zhu	白 朮
Ramulus Cinnamomi	Gui zhi	桂 枝

Energy Tonic Chronic Fatigue (EN-261)

INGREDIENTS

Radix Astragli	Huang qi	黃 耆
Radix Ginseng	Ren shen	人 參
Rhizoma Atrctylodis	Bai zhu	白 朮
Rhizoma Polygonti	Huang jing	黃 精
Radix Angelicae	Dang gui	當 歸
Radix Bupleuri	Chai hu	柴 胡
Rhizoma Cimicifugae	Sheng ma	升 麻
Citri Leiocarpae Exomcarpium	Chen pi	陳 皮
Rhizoma Zingiberis	Sheng jiang	生 姜
Fructus Zizyphi	Da Zao	大 棗
Radix Glycyrrhizae	Gan cao	甘 草

Gastrointestinal Poor Digestion (GI-335)

INGREDIENTS

Fructus Citri Sarcodactyli	Fo shou gan	佛 手 乾
Immaturus Aurantii Fructus	Zhi shi	枳 實
Rhizoma Cyperi	Xiang fu zi	香 附 子
Rhizoma Corydalis Yanhusuo	Yan hu suo	延 胡 索
Rhizoma Rhei	Da huang	大 黃
Fermaentata Massa Medicata	Shen qu	神 曲
Fructus Gardeniae	Zhi zi	梔 子

Gastrointestinal Excess Acid, Ulcer (GI-337)

INGREDIENTS

Rhizoma Coptidis	Huang lian	黃 連
Tuber Pinelliae	Ban xia	半 夏
Cortex Phellodendri	Huang bai	黃 柏
Fructus Evodiae	Wu zhu yu	吳 茱 萸
Immaturus Fructus Aurantii	Zhi shi	枳 實
Rhizoma Rhei	Da huang	大 黃
Caulis in Taeniis Bambussae	Zhu ru	竹 茹
Radix Paeoniae	Shao yao	芍 藥
Concha Cyclina	Hai ge fen	海 蛤 粉

Headache, Migraine, Tension (HA-341)

INGREDIENTS

Rhizoma Ligustici	Chuan xiong	川 芎
Rhizoma Corydalis Yanhusuo	Yan hu suo	延 胡 索
Radix Angelicae Dahuricae	Bai zhi	白 芷
Rhizoma Notoerygii	Qiang huo	羌 活
Radix Angelicae Tuchuo	Du huo	獨 活
Radix Ledebouriellae	Fang feng	防 風
Herba cum Radice Asri	Xixin	細 辛
Fructus Viticis	Man jing zi	蔓 荊 子
Flos Chrysanthemi	Ju hua	菊 花
Radix Angelicae	Dang gui	當 歸
Rhizoma Atractylodis Lanceae	Cang zhu	蒼 朮
Tuber Ophiopogonis	Mai men dong	麥 門 冬
Radix Scutellariae	Huang qin	黃 耆
Rhizoma Zingibeeris Xiccatum	Gan jiang	乾 姜
Radix Glycyrrhizae	Gan cao	甘 草

Hemorrhoids, Constipation (HE-349)

INGREDIENTS

Rhizoma Cimicifugae	Sheng ma	升 麻
Radix Bupleuri	Chai hu	柴 胡
Radix Angelicae	Dang gui	當 歸
Radix Scutellariae	Huang qin	黄 芩
Rhizoma Rhei	Da huang	大 黄
Radix Glycyrrhizae	Gan cao	甘 草

Hypertension High Blood Pressure (HB-345)

INGREDIENTS

Rhizoma Gastrodiae	Tiang ma	天 麻
Ramulus cum Uncus Uncariae	Diao teng gou	吊 藤 鉤
Concha Haliotidis	Shi jue ming	石 決 明
Herba Siegesbeckia	Xi xian cao	豨 薟 草
Fructus Gardeniae	Zhi zi	梔 子
Radix Scutellariae	Huang qin	黄 芩
Herba leonuri	Yi mu cao	益 母 草
Radix Achyranthis	Niu xi	牛 膝
Cortex Eucommiae	Du zhong	杜 仲
Ramulus Loranthi	Sang ji sheng	桑 寄 生
Caulis Polygonum Multiflori	Ye jiao teng	夜 交 藤
Poria Fu ling	Fu ling	茯 苓
Rhizoma Alismatis	Ze xie	澤 瀉

Insomnia, Anxiety (SL-749)

INGREDIENTS

Semen Zizyphi Spinosi	Suan zao ren	酸 棗 仁
Caulis Polygoni Multiflori	Ye jiao teng	夜 交 藤
Cortex Albizziae	He huan pi	合 歡 皮
Poria	Fu ling	茯 苓
Rhizoma Ligustici	Chuan xiong	川 芎
Fructus Schizandrae	Wu wei zi	五 味 子

INGREDIENTS CONTINUED FROM PAGE 232

Rhizoma Coptidis	Huang lian	黄 連
Rhizoma Anemarrhenae	Zhi mu	知 母
Radix Rehmanniae	Di huang	地 黄
Radix Glycyrrhizae	Gan cao	甘 草

Ligament, Connective Tissue Repair (LI-485)

INGREDIENTS

Radix Ginseng	Ren shen	人 參
Rhizoma Atractylodis	Bai zhu	白 芷
Poria	Fu ling	茯 苓
Radix Astragali	Huang qi	黄 芩
Radix Angelicae	Dang gui	當 歸
Radix Rehmanniae	Sheng di huang	生 地 黄
Radix Peoniae	Shao yao	芍 藥
Rhizoma Ligustici	Chuan xiong	川 芎
Ramulus Cinnamomi	Gui zhi	桂 枝
Radix Glycyrrhizae	Gan cao	甘 草

Ligament, Muscle Weakness (LI-487)

INGREDIENTS

Radix Rehmanniae	Sheng di huang	生 地 黄
Fructus Corni	Shan zhu yu	山 茱 萸
Fructus Lycii	Gou qi zi	枸 杞 子
Rhizoma Dioscorea Batatis	Shan yao	山 藥
Semen Cuscutae	Tu si zi	兎 絲 子
Radix Achyranthes	Niu xi	牛 膝
Radix Paeoniae	Shao yao	芍 藥
Cortex Eucommiae	Du zhong	杜 仲
Rhizoma Cibatii	Gou ji	狗 脊

Liver Detoxification (LD-477)

INGREDIENTS		
Radix Bupleri	Chai hu	柴 胡
Radix Angelicae	Dang gui	當 歸
Radix Paeoniae	Shao yao	芍 藥
Rhizoma Ligustici	Chuan xiong	川 芎
Radix Rehmannia	Di huang	地 黄
Radix Scutellariae	Huang qin	黄 芩
Rhizoma Coptidis	Huang lian	黄 連
Cortex Phellodendri	Huang bai	黄 柏
Fructus Gardeniae	Zhi zi	梔 子
Fructus forsythiae	Lian qiao	連 翹
Radix Trichosanthis	Gua lou gen	瓜 蔞 根
Rhizoma Alismatis	Ze xie	澤 瀉
Herba Mathae	Bo he	薄 荷
Fructus Arctii	Niu bang zi	牛 蒡 子
Radix Platycodi	Jie geng	桔 梗
Radix Glycyrrhizae	Gan cao	甘 草

Men's Formula (MA-511)

INGREDIENTS		
Radix Astragali	Huang qi	黄 耆
Radix Ginseng	Ren shen	人 參
Cornu Cervi Colla	Lu jiao jiao	鹿 角 膠
Cortex Eucommiae	Du zhong	杜 仲
Semen Cuscutae	Tu si zi	兔 絲 子
Herba Epimedii	Yin yang huo	淫 羊 藿
Cortex Cinnamomi	Gui pi	桂 皮
Radix Angelicae	Dang gui	當 歸
Radix Rehmanniae	Di huaang	地 黄
Fructus Corni	Shan zhu yu	山 茱 萸
Rhizoma Dioscorea Batatis	Shan yao	山 藥

Pre- and Post Menopause (ME-523)

INGREDIENTS

Radix Ginseng	Ren shen	人 參
Rhizoma Atractylodis	Bai zhu	白 朮
Radix Glycyrrhizae	Gan cao	甘 草
Radix Angelicae	Dang gui	當 歸
Rhizoma Ligustici	Chuan xiong	川 芎
Rhizoma Coptidis	Huang lian	黃 連
Radix Scutellariae	Huang qin	黃 芩
Rhizoma Rhei	Da huang	大 黃
Ramulus Cinnamomi	Gui zhi	桂 枝
Radix Saussureae	Mu xiang	木 香
Semen Arecae	Bing lang zi	檳 榔 子
Rhizoma Cyperi	Xiang fu zi	香 附 子
Flos Caryphyli	Ding xiang	丁 香

Pain Relief Shoulders, Neck, Upper Body (PA-621)

INGREDIENTS

Radix Puerariae	Ge gen	葛 根
Ramulus Cinnamomi	Gui zhi	桂 枝
Radix Paeoniae	Shao yao	芍 藥
Radix Glycyrrhizae	Gan cao	甘 草
Rhizoma Ligustici	Chuan xiong	川 芎
Herba Ephedrae	Ma huang	麻 黃
Rhizoma Notoptergii	Qiang huo	羌 活
Rhizoma Zingiberis Siccatum	Gan jiang	乾 姜
Fructus Zizyphi	Da zao	大 棗

Pain Relief Low Back and Lower Body (PA-623)

INGREDIENTS

Radix Angelicae	Dang gui	當歸
Gummi Olibanum	Ru xiang	乳香
Myrrha	Mo yao	沒藥
Ramulus Cinnamomi	Gui zhi	桂枝
Radix Paeoniae	Shao yao	芍藥
Radix Rehmanniae	Di huang	地黃
Rhizoma Ligustici	Chuan xiong	川芎
Semen Persicae	Tao ren	桃仁
Rhizoma Notopterygii	Qiang huo	羌活
Radix Ledebouriellae	Fang feng	防風
Radix Angelicae Dahuricae	Bai zhi	白芷
Radix Clematidis	Wei ling xian	威靈仙
Radix Aristolochiae Fangchi	Fang ji	防己
Radix Gentiana Scabrae	Long dan cao	龍膽草
Radix Achyranthis	Niu xi	牛膝
Rhizoma Atractylodis	Bai zhu	白朮
Poria	Fu ling	茯苓
Exocarpium Citri Leiocarpae	Chen pi	陳皮
Rhizoma Zingiberis	Sheng jiang	生姜
Radix Glycyrrhizae	Gan cao	甘草

Premenstrual Formula

INGREDIENTS

Radix Bupleuri	Chai hu	柴胡
Radix Angelicae	Dang gui	當歸
Radix Paeoniae	Shao yao	芍藥
Rhizoma Atractylodis	Bai zhu	白芷
Poria	Fu ling	茯苓
Herba Menthae	Bo he	薄荷
Cortex Moutasn Radicis	Mu dan pi	牡丹皮
Fructus Gardeniae	Zhi zi	梔子
Radix Glycyrrhizae	Gan cao	甘草
Rhizoma Zingiberis siccatum	Gan jiang	乾姜

Premenstrual Formula (PM-637)

INGREDIENTS

Semen Persicae	Tao ren	桃 仁
Cortex Moutan Racicis	Mu dan pi	牡 丹 皮
Radix Rehmanniae	Sheng di huang	生 地 黄
Fructus Corni	Shan zhu yu	山 茱 萸
Rhizoma Dioscorea Batatis	Shan yao	山 藥
Poria	Fu ling	茯 苓
Rhizoma Alismatis	Ze xie	澤 瀉
Semen Coicis	Yi yi ren	薏 苡 仁
Ramulus Cinnamomi	Gui zhi	桂 枝
Rhizoma Rhei	Da huang	大 黄
Sulfuricum Natrium	Mang xiao	芒 硝
Semen Benincasae	Dong gua zi	冬 瓜 子
Rhizoma Atractylodis Lanceae	Cang zhu	蒼 朮
Radix Glycyrrhizae	Gan cao	甘 草

Sinus Infection, Congestion (NA-551)

INGREDIENTS

Radix Puerariae	Ge gen	葛 根
Herba Ephedrae	Ma huang	麻 黄
Flos Magnoliae Liliflora	Xin yi	辛 荑
Herba Houttuyniae	Yu xing cao	魚 腥 草
Radix Angelicae Dahuricae	Bai zhi	白 芷
Ramulus Cinnammomi	Gui zhi	桂 枝
Radix Peoniae	Shao yao	芍 藥
Rhizoma Ligustici	Chuan xiong	川 芎
Rhizoma Zingiberis	Sheng jiang	生 姜
Fructus Zizyphi	Da zao	大 棗
Radix Glycyrrhizae	Gan cao	甘 草

Stress Relief, Anxiety (RE-699)

INGREDIENTS		
Radix Bupleuri	Chai hu	柴 胡
Radix Scutellariae	Huang qin	黃 芩
Ramulus Cinnamomi	Gui zhi	桂 枝
Rhizoma Rhei	Da huang	大 黃
Os Draconis	Long gu	龍 骨
Testa Ostraea	Mu li	牡 蠣
Radix Ginseng	Ren shen	人 參
Poria	Fu ling	茯 苓
Tuber Pinelliae	Ban xia	半 夏
Rhizoma Zingiberis	Sheng jiang	生 姜
Fructus Zizyphi	Da zao	大 棗

Skin Eruptions and Acne (SK-741)

INGREDIENTS		
Flos Lonicerae	Jin yin hua	金 銀 花
Fructus Gardeniae	Zhi zi	梔 子
Fructus Forsythiae	Lian qiao	連 翹
Herba Taraxaci	Pu gong ying	蒲 公 英
Herba Vioae	Zi hua di ding	紫 花 地 丁
Radix Glycyrrhizae	Gan cao	甘 草
Radix Scutellariae	Huang qin	黃 芩
Radix Sophorae	Ku shen	苦 參
Radix Paeoniae Rubra	Chi shao	赤 芍
Cortex Moutan Radixis	Mu dan pi	牡 丹 皮
Radix Rehmannia	Di huang	地 黃
Radix Angelicae Dahuricae	Bai zhi	白 芷
Radix Platycodi	Jiegeng	桔 梗
Radix Ledebouriellae	Fang feng	防 風
Semen Coicis Semen	Yi yi ren	薏 苡 仁

Trauma, Injury (TR-797)

INGREDIENTS

Radix Angelicae	Dang gui	當 歸
Gummi Olibanum	Ru xiang	乳 香
Myrrha	Mo yao	沒 藥
Semen Persicae	Tao ren	桃 仁
Flos Carthami	Hong hua	紅 花
Rhizoma Rhei	Da huang	大 黃
Rhizoma Ligustici	Chuan xiong	川 芎
Radix Notoginseng	San qi	三 七
Radix Trichosanthes	Gua lou gen	瓜 蔞 根
Radix Bupleuri	Chai hu	柴 胡
Radix Glycyrrhizae	Gan cao	甘 草

Urinary Tract Infections (UI-821)

INGREDIENTS

Herba Dianthi	Qu mai	瞿 麥
Caulis Akebiae	Mu tong	木 通
Herba Polygoni Aviculari	Bian xu	萹 蓄
Semen Plantaginis	Che qian zi	車 前 子
Talcum and Kaolinum	Hua shi	滑 石
Medulla Junci Caulis	Deng xin cao	燈 芯 草
Fructus Gardiniae	Zhi zi	梔 子
Rhizoma Rhei	Da huang	大 黃
Radix Glycyrrhizae	Gan cao	甘 草

THE THREE TREASURES

Bend Bamboo

INGREDIENTS

Radix Angelicae Sinensis	Dang gui	當 歸
Radix Ligustici Wallichii	Chuan xiong	川 芎
Radix Rehmanniae Glutinosae Conquitae	Shu di huang	熟 地 黄
Ramus Loranthi seu Visci	Sang ji sheng	桑 寄 生
Radix Paeoniae Lactiflorae	Bai shao	白 芍
Flos Chrysanthemi Morifolii	Ju hua	菊 花
Rhizoma Gastrodiae Elatae	Tian ma	天 麻
Fructus Viticis	Man jing zi	蔓 荆 子
Fructus Tribuli Terrestris	Bai ji li	白 蒺 藜
Fructus Lycii Chinensis	Gou qi zi	枸 杞 子
Sclerotium Poriae Cocos	Fu ling	茯 苓
Radix Glycyrrhizae Uralensis	Zhi gan cao	炙 甘 草

Break Into a Smile

INGREDIENTS

Radix Bupleuri	Chai hu	柴 胡
Radix Paeoniae Lactiflorae	Bai shao	白 芍
Radix Glycyrrhizae Uralensis	Zhi gan cao	炙 甘 草
Fructus Citri Aurantii	Zhi ke	枳 殼
Percarpium citri Reticulatae	Chen pi	陳 皮
Rhizoma Cyperi Rotundi	Xiang fu	香 附
Radix Ligustici Wallichii	Chuan xiong	川 芎
Radix Salviae Miltiorrhizae	Dan shen	丹 參
Radix Pseudostellariae Heterophyllae	Tai zi shen	太 子 參
Rhizoma Corydalis	Yan hu suo	延 胡 索
Semen Zizyphi Spinosae	Suan zao ren	酸 棗 仁
Sclerotium Poriae Cocos	Fu ling	茯 苓

Brighten the Eyes

INGREDIENTS

Radix Angelicae Sinensis	Dang gui	當 歸
Radix Rehmanniae Glutinosae Conquitae	Shu di huang	熟 地 黃
Radix Ligustici Wallichii	Chuan xiong	川 芎
Radix Paeoniae Lactiflorae	Bai shao	白 芍
Fructus Lycii Chinensis	Gou qi zi	枸 杞 子
Semen Cuscutae	Tu si zi	兔 絲 子
Frutus Ligustri Lucidi	Nu zhen zi	女 貞 子
Flos Chrysanthemi Morifolii	Ju hua	菊 花
Fructus Viticis	Man jing zi	蔓 荆 子
Buddliea Officinalis	Mi meng hua	密 蒙 花
Fructus Tribuli Terrestris	Bai ji li	白 蒺 藜
Radix Polygoni Multiflori	Shou wu	首 烏
Fructus Zizyphi Jujubae	Hong zao	紅 棗

Calm the Spirit

INGREDIENTS

Radix Ginseng	Ren shen	人 參
Radix Astragali	Huang qi	黃 耆
Radix Angelicae Sinensis	Dang gui	當 歸
Sclerotium Poriae Cocos	Fu shen	茯 神
Semen Zizyphi Spinosae	Suan zao ren	酸 棗 仁
Arillus Euphoriae Longanae	Long yan rou	龍 眼 肉
Radix Polygale Tenuifoliae Recens	Yuan zhi	遠 志
Radix Saussureae seu Vladimiriae	Mu xiang	木 香
Radix Glycyrrhizae Uralensis	Zhi gan cao	炙 甘 草
Fructus Zizyphi Jujubae	Hong zao	紅 棗
Semen Biotae Orientalis	Bai zi ren	柏 子 仁
Cortex Albizziae Julibrissin	He huan pi	合 歡 皮
Rhizoma Acori Graminei	Shi chang pu	石 菖 蒲
Bulbus Lilii	Bai he	百 合

Central Mansion

INGREDIENTS

Radix Ginseng	Ren shen	人 參
Rhizoma Atractylodis Macrocephalae	Bai zhu	白 朮
Sclerotium Poriae Cocos	Fu ling	茯 苓
Radix Glycyrrhizae Uralensis	Zhi gan cao	炙 甘 草
Semen Dolichoris	Bai bian dou	白 扁 豆
Radix Dioscoreae Oppositae	Shan yao	山 藥
Semen Nelumbins	Lian zi	蓮 子
Fructus seu Semen Amomi	Sha ren	砂 仁
Semen Coicis	Yi yi ren	薏 苡 仁
Radix Platycodi Grandiflori	Jie geng	桔 梗
Radix Pseudostellariae Heterophyllae	Tai zi shen	太 子 參
Rhizoma Polygonati Odorati	Yu zhu	玉 竹
Radix Panacis Quinquefolii	Xi yang shen	西 洋 參

Clear Lustre

INGREDIENTS

Radix Polygoni Multiflori	Shou wu	首 烏
Radix Angelicae Sinensis	Dang gui	當 歸
Cortex Dictamni Radicis	Bai xian pi	白 蘚 皮
Radix Ledebouriellae Sesloidis	Fang feng	防 風
Herba seu Flos Schizonepetae Tenuifoliae	Jing jie	荊 芥
Flos Chrysanthemi Morifolii	Ju hua	菊 花
Radix Sophorae Flavescentis	Ku shen	苦 參
Cortex Moutan Radicis	Mu dan pi	牡 丹 皮
Radix Scutellariae Baicalensis	Huang qin	黃 芩
Gypsum	Shi gao	石 膏
Radix Anemarrhenae	Zhi mu	知 母
Radix Glycyrrhizae Uralensis	Gan cao	甘 草

Clear Qi

INGREDIENTS

Fructus Perillae Frutescentis	Su zi	蘇 子
Rhizoma Pinelliae Ternatae	Ban xia	半 夏
Cortex Magnoliae Officinalis	Hou po	厚 樸
Radix Peucedaani	Qian hu	前 胡
Cortex Cinnamomi Cassiae	Rou gui	肉 桂
Radix Angelicae Sinensis	Dang gui	當 歸
Flos Inulae	Xuan fu hua	旋 复 花
Lignum Aquilariae	Chen xiang	沉 香
Semen Pruni Armeniacae	Ku xing ren	苦 杏 仁
Radix Asteris Tatarici	Zi wan	紫 苑
Radix Ledebouriellae Sesloidis	Fang feng	防 風
Folium Mori Albae	Sang ye	桑 葉
Cortex Mori Albae Raicis	Sang bai pi	桑 白 皮
Frutus Schisandrae Chinensis	Wu wei zi	五 味 子
Radix Salviae Miltiorrhizae	Dan shen	丹 參
Semen Juglandis	Hu tao rou	胡 桃 肉
Radix Scutellariae Baicalensis	Huang qin	黃 芩
Radix Glycyrrhizae Uralensis	Zhi gan cao	炙 甘 草

Clear the Root

INGREDIENTS

Radix Astragali	Huang qi	黃 耆
Cortex Cinnamomi Cassiae	Rou gui	肉 桂
Radix Rehmanniae	Sheng di huang	生 地 黃
Radix Anemarrhenae	Zhi mu	知 母
Cortex Phellodendri	Huang bai	黃 柏
Frutus Ligustri Lucidi	Nu zhen zi	女 貞 子
Semen Cuscutae	Tu si zi	兎 絲 子
Radix Dioscoreae Oppositae	Shan yao	山 藥
Sclerotium Poriae Cocos	Fu ling	茯 苓
Rhizoma Alismatis Plantago-aquaticae	Ze xie	澤 瀉
Semen Coicis	Yi yi ren	薏 苡 仁

Semen Plantaginis	Che qian zi	車前子
Rhizoma Dioscoreae Hypogloaucae	Bei xie	萆薢
Semen Persicae	Tao ren	桃仁
Semen Vaccariae Segetalis	Wang bu liu xing	王不留行
Cortex Moutan Radicis	Mu dan pi	牡丹皮
Rhizoma Acori Graminei	Shi chang pu	石菖莆
Herba Hedyotidis Diffusae	Bai hua she she cao	白花蛇舌草
Radix Glycyrrhizae Uralensis	Gan cao	甘草

Clear the Soul

INGREDIENTS

Caulis Bambusae in Taeniis	Zhu ru	竹茹
Fructus Immaturus Citri Aurantii	Zhi shi	枳實
Rhizoma Pinelliae Ternatae	Ban xia	半夏
Sclerotium Poriae Cocos	Fu ling	茯苓
Percarpium citri Reticulatae	Chen pi	陳皮
Fructus Zizyphi Jujubae	Da zao	大棗
Radix Glycyrrhizae Uralensis	Gan cao	甘草
Cortex Albizziae Julibrissin	He huan pi	合歡皮
Tuber Curcumae	Yu jin	郁金
Radix Polygale Tenuifoliae Recens	Yuan zhi	遠志
Rhizoma Acori Graminei	Shi chang pu	石菖莆
Semen Biotae Orientalis	Bai zi ren	柏子仁
Radix Salviae Miltiorrhizae	Dan shen	丹參

Clear Yang

INGREDIENTS

Pinelliae Ternatae	Ban xia	半夏
Rhizoma Gastrodiae Elatae	Tian ma	天麻
Rhizoma Atractylodis Macrocephalae	Bai zhu	白朮
Sclerotium Poriae Cocos	Fu ling	茯苓
Percarpium citri Reticulatae	Chen pi	陳皮
Radix Glycyrrhizae Uralensis	Gan cao	甘草

INGREDIENTS CONTINUED FROM PAGE 244

Fructus Zizyphi Jujubae	Da zao	大棗
Ramulus Uncariae	Gou teng	鉤藤
Fructus Tribuli Terrestris	Bai ji li	白蒺藜
Flos Chrysanthemi Morifolii	Ju hua	菊花
Fructus Viticis	Man jing zi	蔓荊子
Radix Angelicae Sinensis	Dang gui	當歸
Semen Cuscutae	Tu si zi	菟絲子
Cortex Eucommiae Ulmoidis	Du zhong	杜仲
Fructus Lycii Chinensis	Gou qi zi	枸杞子
Radix Polygale Tenuifoliae Recens	Yuan zhi	遠志
Rhizoma Acori Graminei	Shi chang pu	石菖蒲

Chemo Support

INGREDIENTS

Radix Astragali	Huang qi	黄耆
Radix Codonopsis Pilosulae	Dang shen	黨參
Radix Pseudostellariae Heterophyllae	Tai zi shen	太子參
Sclerotium Ganodermae	Ling zhi	靈芝
Radix Dioscoreae Oppositae	Shan yao	山藥
Radix Panacis Quinquefolii	Xi yang shen	西洋參
Cortex Moutan Radicis	Mu dan pi	牡丹皮
Sclerotium Poriae Cocos	Fu ling	茯苓
Percarpium citri Reticulatae	Chen pi	陳皮
Tuber Ophiopogonis Japonici	Mai men dong	麥門冬
Radix Angelicae Sinensis	Dang gui	當歸
Rhizoma Pinelliae Ternatae	Ban xia	半夏
Rhizoma Phragmitis Communis	Lu gen	蘆根
Frutus Ligustri Lucidi	Nu zhen zi	女貞子
Rhizoma Polygonati	Huang jing	黄精
Radix Glycyrrhizae Uralensis	Gan cao	甘草

Children's Herbal Sentinel

INGREDIENTS

Ramulus Cinnamomi	Gui zhi	桂 枝
Radix Paeoniae Lactiflorae	Bai shao	白 芍
Rhizoma Zingiberis Officinalis Recens	Sheng jiang	生 姜
Fructus Zizyphi Jujubae	Da zao	大 棗
Radix Glycyrrhizae Uralensis	Zhi gan cao	炙 甘 草
Massa Fermentata	Shen qu	神 曲
Semen Paphani Sativi	Lai fu zi	萊 菔 子
Fructus Crataegi	Shan zha	山 楂
Fructus Hordei Vulgaris Germinantus	Mai ya	麥 芽
Endothelium Corneum Gigeriae Galli	Ji nei jin	雞 內 金
Radix Pseudostellariae Heterophyllae	Tai zi shen	太 子 參
Radix Astragali	Huang qi	黄 耆
Rhizoma Atractylodis Macrocephalae	Bai zhu	白 朮
Radix Ledebouriellae Sesloidis	Fang feng	防 風
Sclerotium Poriae Cocos	Fu ling	茯 苓
Percarpium citri Reticulatae	Chen pi	陳 皮

Drain Fields

INGREDIENTS

Herba Angastache seu Pogostemi	Huo xiang	藿 香
Rhizoma Pinelliae Ternatae	Ban xia	半 夏
Sclerotium Poriae Cocos	Fu ling	茯 苓
Semen Pruni Armeniacae	Ku xing ren	苦 杏 仁
Semen Coicis	Yi yi ren	薏 苡 仁
Fructus Amonum	Bai dou kou	白 豆 蔻
Sclerotium Polypori Umbellati	Zhu ling	豬 苓
Semen Sojae Praeparatum	Dan dou chi	淡 豆 豉
Rhizoma Alismatis Plantago-aquaticae	Ze xie	澤 瀉
Cortex Magnoliae Officinalis	Hou po	厚 樸
Radix Glycyrrhizae Uralensis	Zhi gan cao	炙 甘 草
Radix Astragali	Huang qi	黄 耆
Rhizoma Atractylodis Macrocephalae	Bai zhu	白 朮

Fructus seu Semen Amomi	Sha ren	砂仁
Herba Eupatorii	Pei lan	佩蘭
Rhizoma Phragmitis Communis	Lu gen	蘆根

Drain Fire

INGREDIENTS

Radix Gentianae Scabrae	Long dan cao	龍膽草
Radix Scutellariae Baicalensis	Huang qin	黃芩
Fructus Gardiniae Jasminoidis	Shan zhi zi	山梔子
Rhizoma Alismatis Plantago-aquaticae	Ze xie	澤瀉
Medulla Tetrapanacis	Tong cao	通草
Semen Plantaginis	Che qian zi	車前子
Radix Rehmanniae	Sheng di huang	生地黄
Radix Angelicae Sinensis	Dang gui	當歸
Radix Bupleuri	Chai hu	柴胡
Radix Glycyrrhizae Uralensis	Gan cao	甘草
Semen Zizyphi Spinosae	Suan zao ren	酸棗仁
Radix Polygale Tenuifoliae Recens	Yuan zhi	遠志
Rhizoma Gastrodiae Elatae	Tian ma	天麻
Flos Chrysanthemi Morifolii	Ju hua	菊花
Ramulus Uncariae	Gou teng	鉤藤
Herba Lophatheri Gracilis	Dan zhu ye	淡竹葉
Plumus Nelumbinis	Lian xin	蓮心

Ease the Journey—Yin

INGREDIENTS

Radix Rehmanniae	Sheng di huang	生地黄
Radix Dioscoreae Oppositae	Shan yao	山藥
Fructus Corni Officinalis	Shan zhu yu	山茱萸
Fructus Lycii Chinensis	Gou qi zi	枸杞子
Semen Cuscutae	Tu si zi	兎絲子
Cornu Cervi Degelatinatium	Lu jiao shuang	鹿角霜

Gelatinum Plastri Testudinis	Gui ban jiao	龜板膠
Radix Glycyrrhizae Uralensis	Zhi gan cao	炙甘草
Rhizoma Alismatis Plantago-aquaticae	Ze xie	澤瀉
Radix Gentianae Macrophyllae	Qin jiao	秦艽
Tuber Asparagi Cochinchinensis	Tian men dong	天門冬
Cortex Moutan Radicis	Mu dan pi	牡丹皮
Cortex Lycii Radicis	Di gu pi	地骨皮
Concha Ostreae	Mu li	牡蠣
Semen Zizyphi Spinosae	Suan zao ren	酸棗仁

Ease the Journey—Yang

INGREDIENTS

Radix Dioscoreae Oppositae	Shan yao	山藥
Radix Rehmanniae	Sheng di huang	生地黄
Fructus Corni Officinalis	Shan zhu yu	山茱萸
Fructus Lycii Chinensis	Gou qi zi	枸杞子
Cornu Cervi Degelatinatium	Lu jiao shuang	鹿角霜
Semen Cuscutae	Tu si zi	兎絲子
Cortex Eucommiae Ulmoidis	Du zhong	杜仲
Radix Angelicae Sinensis	Dang gui	當歸
Cortex Cinnamomi Cassiae	Rou gui	肉桂
Radix Glycyrrhizae Uralensis	Zhi gan cao	炙甘草
Radix Anemarrhenae	Zhi mu	知母
Concha Ostreae	Mu li	牡蠣
Radix Gentianae Macrophyllae	Qin jiao	秦艽
Cortex Lycii Radicis	Di gu pi	地骨皮

Ease the Muscles

INGREDIENTS

Rhizoma Coptidis	Huang lian	黄連
Cortex Magnoliae Officinalis	Hou po	厚樸
Rhizoma Acori Graminei	Shi chang pu	石菖蒲
Rhizoma Pinelliae Ternatae	Ban xia	半夏
Semen Sojae Praeparatum	Dan dou chi	淡豆豉
Fructus Gardiniae Jasminoidis	Shan zhi zi	山梔子
Rhizoma Phragmitis Communis	Lu gen	蘆根
Radix Astragali	Huang qi	黄耆
Rhizoma Atractylodis Macrocephalae	Bai zhu	白朮
Fructus seu Semen Amomi	Sha ren	砂仁
Semen Coicis	Yi yi ren	薏苡仁
Herba Angastache seu Pogostemi	Huo xiang	藿香
Sclerotium Poriae Cocos	Fu ling	茯苓

Expel Wind—Heat

INGREDIENTS

Herba Menthae	Bo he	薄荷
Semen Sojae Praeparatum	Dan dou chi	淡豆豉
Radix Ledebouriellae Sesloidis	Fang feng	防風
Herba Lophatheri Gracilis	Dan zhu ye	淡竹葉
Herba seu Flos Schizonepetae Tenuifoliae	Jing jie	荆芥
Flos Lonicerae Japonicae	Jin yin hua	金銀花
Fructus Forsythiae Suspensae	Lian qiao	連翹
Radix Platycodi Grandiflori	Jie geng	桔梗
Radix Glycyrrhizae Uralensis	Gan cao	甘草
Fructus Arctii Lappae	Niu bang zi	牛蒡子
Folium Daqingye	Da qing ye	大青葉
Flos Chrysanthemi Morifolii	Ju hua	菊花
Semen Pruni Armeniacae	Ku xing ren	苦杏仁
Radix Scutellariae Baicalensis	Huang qin	黄芩

Freeing the Moon

INGREDIENTS

Radix Bupleuri	Chai hu	柴 胡
Herba Menthae	Bo he	薄 荷
Radix Angelicae Sinensis	Dang gui	當 歸
Radix Paeoniae Lactiflorae	Bai shao	白 芍
Radix Codonopsis Pilosulae	Dang shen	黨 參
Sclerotium Poriae Cocos	Fu ling	茯 苓
Fructus Lycii Chinensis	Gou qi zi	枸 杞 子
Radix Polygoni Multiflori	Shou wu	首 烏
Pericarpium Citri Reticulatae Viride	Qing pi	青 皮
Cortex Albizziae Julibrissin	He huan pi	合 歡 皮
Radix Polygale Tenuifoliae Recens	Yuan zhi	遠 志
Bulbus Lilii	Bai he	百 合
Radix Glycyrrhizae Uralensis	Gan cao	甘 草
Fructus Zizyphi Jujubae	Hong zao	紅 棗
Flos Chrysanthemi Morifolii	Ju hua	菊 花

Glorious Sea

INGREDIENTS

Radix Angelicae Sinensis	Dang gui	當 歸
Radix Polygoni Multiflori	Shou wu	首 烏
Fructus Lycii Chinensis	Gou qi zi	枸 杞 子
Cortex Dictamni Radicis	Bai xian pi	白 蘚 皮
Semen Cuscutae	Tu si zi	兎 絲 子
Radix Rehmanniae	Sheng di huang	生 地 黄
Rhizoma Alismatis Plantago-aquaticae	Ze xie	澤 瀉
Rhizoma Pinelliae Ternatae	Ban xia	半 夏
Sclerotium Poriae Cocos	Fu ling	茯 苓
Radix Glycyrrhizae Uralensis	Gan cao	甘 草
Radix Scutellariae Baicalensis	Huang qin	黄 芩
Cortex Moutan Radicis	Mu dan pi	牡 丹 皮

Herbal Sentinel—Yang

INGREDIENTS

Radix Astragali	Huang qi	黄 耆
Radix Ginseng	Ren shen	人 參
Sclerotium Ganodermae	Ling zhi	靈 芝
Rhizoma Atractylodis Macrocephalae	Bai zhu	白 朮
Radix Ledebouriellae Sesloidis	Fang feng	防 風
Ramulus Cinnamomi	Gui zhi	桂 枝
Radix Paeoniae Lactiflorae	Bai shao	白 芍
Rhizoma Zingiberis Officinalis Recens	Sheng jiang	生 姜
Fructus Zizyphi Jujubae	Da zao	大 棗
Radix Glycyrrhizae Uralensis	Zhi gan cao	炙 甘 草
Semen Cuscutae	Tu si zi	兎 絲 子
Cornu Cervi Degelatinatium	Lu jiao shuang	鹿 角 霜
Radix Morindae Officinalis	Ba ji tian	巴 戟 天
Frutus Schisandrae Chinensis	Wu wei zi	五 味 子
Sclerotium Poriae Cocos	Fu ling	茯 苓
Radix Scutellariae Baicalensis	Huang qin	黄 芩
Rhizoma Polygonati Odorati	Yu zhu	玉 竹

Herbal Sentinel—Yin

INGREDIENTS

Radix Astragali	Huang qi	黄 耆
Radix Panacis Quinquefolii	Xi yang shen	西 洋 參
Sclerotium Ganodermae	Ling zhi	靈 芝
Frutus Schisandrae Chinensis	Wu wei zi	五 味 子
Tuber Ophiopogonis Japonici	Mai men dong	麥 門 冬
Radix Glehniae	Bei sha shen	北 沙 參
Bulbus Lilii	Bai he	百 合
Rhizoma Polygonati Odorati	Yu zhu	玉 竹
Radix Rehmanniae Glutinosae Conquitae	Shu di huang	熟 地 黄
Fructus Corni Officinalis	Shan zhu yu	山 茱 萸
Radix Dioscoreae Oppositae	Shan yao	山 藥
Fructus Zizyphi Jujubae	Da zao	大 棗

Radix Glycyrrhizae Uralensis	Zhi gan cao	炙 甘 草
Radix Anemarrhenae	Zhi mu	知 母
Sclerotium Poriae Cocos	Fu ling	茯 苓

Jade Screen

INGREDIENTS

Fructus Xanthii Sivirici	Cang er zi	蒼 耳 子
Flos Magnoliae liliflor	Xin yi hua	辛 夷 花
Radix Ledebouriellae Sesloidis	Fang feng	防 風
Radix Astragali	Huang qi	黄 耆
Rhizoma Atractylodis Macrocephalae	Bai zhu	白 朮
Radix Angelicae	Bai zhi	白 芷
Fructus Pruni Mume	Wu mei	烏 梅
Frutus Schisandrae Chinensis	Wu wei zi	五 味 子
Radix Salviae Miltiorrhizae	Dan shen	丹 參
Herba Agastaches seu Pogostemi	Hou xiang	藿 香
Herba Menthae	Bo he	薄 荷
Fructus Viticis	Man jing zi	蔓 荆 子
Herba seu Flos Schizonepetae Tenuifoliae	Jing jie	荆 芥
Radix Scutellariae Baicalensis	Huang qin	黄 芩
Radix Glycyrrhizae Uralensis	Gan cao	甘 草
Radix Peucedaani	Qian hu	前 胡
Radix et Rhizoma Cynanchi Baiqian	Bai qian	白 前

Jade Spring

INGREDIENTS

Radix Glehniae	Bei sha shen	北 沙 參
Tuber Ophiopogonis Japonici	Mai men dong	麥 門 冬
Rhizoma Polygonati Odorati	Yu zhu	玉 竹
Radix Glycyrrhizae Uralensis	Gan cao	甘 草
Folium Mori Albae	Sang ye	桑 葉
Semen Dolichoris	Bai bian dou	白 扁 豆
Radix Trichosanthis Kirilowii	Tian hua fen	天 花 粉

INGREDIENTS CONTINUED FROM PAGE 252

Herba Dendrobii	Shi hu	石 斛
Radix Pseudostellariae Heterophyllae	Tai zi shen	太 子 參
Radix Codonopsis Pilosulae	Dang shen	黨 參
Sclerotium Poriae Cocos	Fu ling	茯 苓
Radix Anemarrhenae	Zhi mu	知 母
Radix Dioscoreae Oppositae	Shan yao	山 藥

Limpid Sea

INGREDIENTS

Rhizoma Pinelliae Ternatae	Ban xia	半 夏
Sclerotium Poriae Cocos	Fu ling	茯 苓
Percarpium citri Reticulatae	Chen pi	陳 皮
Radix Glycyrrhizae Uralensis	Gan cao	甘 草
Fructus Zizyphi Jujubae	Da zao	大 棗
Fructus Pruni Mume	Wu mei	烏 梅
Caulis Bambusae in Taeniis	Zhu ru	竹 茹
Fructus Trichosanthis	Gua lou	瓜 蔞
Rhizoma Zingiberis Officinalis	Gan jiang	乾 姜

Nourish the Root

INGREDIENTS

Radix Rehmanniae Glutinosae Conquitae	Shu di huang	熟 地 黄
Radix Dioscoreae Oppositae	Shan yao	山 藥
Fructus Corni Officinalis	Shan zhu yu	山 茱 萸
Fructus Lycii Chinensis	Gou qi zi	枸 杞 子
Radix Achyranthis Bidentatae	Huai niu xi	淮 牛 膝
Semen Cuscutae	Tu si zi	兎 絲 子
Cornu Cervi Degelatinatium	Lu jiao shuang	鹿 角 霜
Gelatinum Plastri Testudinis	Gui ban jiao	龜 板 膠
Radix Glycyrrhizae Uralensis	Zhi gan cao	炙 甘 草
Rhizoma Alismatis Plantago-aquaticae	Ze xie	澤 瀉
Tuber Asparagi Cochinchinensis	Tian men dong	天 門 冬
Cortex Lycii Radicis	Di gu pi	地 骨 皮

Nourish the Root and Clear Wind

INGREDIENTS

Radix Rehmanniae Glutinosae Conquitae	Shu di huang	熟地黄
Radix Rehmanniae	Sheng di huang	生地黄
Rhizoma Polygonati Odorati	Yu zhu	玉竹
Radix Paeoniae Lactiflorae	Bai shao	白芍
Cortex Moutan Radicis	Mu dan pi	牡丹皮
Radix Anemarrhenae	Zhi mu	知母
Cortex Acanthopanacis Gracilistyli Radiis	Wu jia pi	五加皮
Fructus Chaenomelis	Mu gua	木瓜
Ramus Loranthi seu Visci	Sang ji sheng	桑寄生
Radix Gentianae Macrophyllae	Qin jiao	秦艽
Radix Clematis	Wei ling xian	威靈仙
Herba Siegesbeckia	Xi xian cao	豨薟草
Caulis Piperis Kadsurae	Hai feng teng	海風藤
Radix Glycyrrhizae Uralensis	Zhi gan cao	炙甘草

Open the Heart

INGREDIENTS

Rhizoma Pinelliae Ternatae	Ban xia	半夏
Cortex Magnoliae Officinalis	Hou po	厚樸
Folium Perillae Frutescentis	Zi su ye	紫蘇葉
Fructus Zizyphi Jujubae	Da zao	大棗
Radix Glycyrrhizae Uralensis	Gan cao	甘草
Radix Bupleuri	Chai hu	柴胡
Bulbus Lilii	Bai he	百合
Radix Platycodi Grandiflori	Jie geng	桔梗
Pericarpium Citri Reticulatae Viride	Qing pi	青皮
Cortex Albizziae Julibrissin	He huan pi	合歡皮

Peaceful Sunset

INGREDIENTS

Radix Gentianae Scabrae	Long dan cao	龍 膽 草
Rhizoma Gastrodiae Elatae	Tian ma	天 麻
Ramulus Uncariae	Gou teng	鉤 藤
Bulbus Fritillariae Thunbergii	Zhe bei mu	浙 貝 母
Caulis Bambusae in Taeniis	Zhu ru	竹 茹
Fructus Trichosanthis	Gua lou	瓜 蔞
Rhizoma Pinelliae Ternatae	Ban xia	半 夏
Sclerotium Poriae Cocos	Fu ling	茯 苓
Percarpium citri Reticulatae	Chen pi	陳 皮
Flos Chrysanthemi Morifolii	Ju hua	菊 花
Fructus Tribuli Terrestris	Bai ji li	白 蒺 藜
Cortex Moutan Radicis	Mu dan pi	牡 丹 皮
Radix Paeoniae	Chi shao	赤 芍
Caulis Polygoni Multiflori	Ye jiao teng	夜 交 藤
Radix Rehmanniae	Sheng di huang	生 地 黄
Radix Glycyrrhizae Uralensis	Gan cao	甘 草

Radio-Support

INGREDIENTS

Radix Astragali	Huang qi	黄 耆
Radix Angelicae Sinensis	Dang gui	當 歸
Flos Carthami Tinctorii	Hong hua	紅 花
Radix Salviae Miltiorrhizae	Dan shen	丹 參
Radix Pseudostellariae Heterophyllae	Tai zi shen	太 子 參
Radix Polygoni Multiflori	Shou wu	首 烏
Fructus Lycii Chinensis	Gou qi zi	枸 杞 子
Frutus Schisandrae Chinensis	Wu wei zi	五 味 子
Frutus Ligustri Lucidi	Nu zhen zi	女 貞 子
Radix Anemarrhenae	Zhi mu	知 母
Cortex Moutan Radicis	Mu dan pi	牡 丹 皮
Radix Paeoniae	Chi shao	赤 芍
Radix Glycyrrhizae Uralensis	Gan cao	甘 草

Red Stirring

INGREDIENTS

Radix Angelicae Sinensis	Dang gui	當 歸
Radix Rehmanniae	Sheng di huang	生 地 黄
Radix Ligustici Wallichii	Chuan xiong	川 芎
Radix Paeoniae	Chi shao	赤 芍
Semen Persicae	Tao ren	桃 仁
Flos Carthami Tinctorii	Hong hua	紅 花
Radix Bupleuri	Chai hu	柴 胡
Fructus Citri Aurantii	Zhi ke	枳 殼
Radix Achyranthis Bidentatae	Niu xi	牛 膝
Radix Platycodi Grandiflori	Jie geng	桔 梗
Radix Glycyrrhizae Uralensis	Gan cao	甘 草
Radix Salviae Miltiorrhizae	Dan shen	丹 參
Radix Polygale Tenuifoliae Recens	Yuan zhi	遠 志
Tuber Curcumae	Yu jin	郁 金
Cortex Albizziae Julibrissin	He huan pi	合 歡 皮

Release Constraint

INGREDIENTS

Rhizoma Cyperi Rotundi	Xiang fu	香 附
Radix Ligustici Wallichii	Chuan xiong	川 芎
Rhizoma Atractyloidis	Cang zhu	蒼 朮
Fructus Gardiniae Jasminoidis	Shan zhi zi	山 梔 子
Massa Fermentata	Shen qu	神 曲
Cortex Albizziae Julibrissin	He huan pi	合 歡 皮
Rhizoma Acori Graminei	Shi chang pu	石 菖 蒲
Radix Glycyrrhizae Uralensis	Gan cao	甘 草

Root the Spirit

INGREDIENTS

Radix Paeoniae Lactiflorae	Bai shao	白芍
Radix Angelicae Sinensis	Dang gui	當歸
Os Draconis	Long gu	龍骨
Semen Cuscutae	Tu si zi	兔絲子
Tuber Ophiopogonis Japonici	Mai men dong	麥門冬
Semen Biotae Orientalis	Bai zi ren	柏子仁
Semen Zizyphi Spinosae	Suan zao ren	酸棗仁
Sclerotium Poriae Cocos	Fu shen	茯神

Separate Clear and Turbid

INGREDIENTS

Rhizoma Dioscoreae Hypogloaucae	Bei xie	萆薢
Radix Linderae Strychnifoliae	Wu yao	烏藥
Fructus Alpiniae Oxyphyllae	Yi zhi ren	益智仁
Rhizoma Acori Graminei	Shi chang pu	石菖蒲
Sclerotium Poriae Cocos	Fu ling	茯苓
Radix Glycyrrhizae Uralensis	Gan cao	甘草
Radix Astragali	Huang qi	黃耆
Semen Plantaginis	Che qian zi	車前子
Herba Dianthi	Qu mai	瞿麥
Radix Paeoniae Lactiflorae	Bai shao	白芍
Radix Morindae Officinalis	Ba ji tian	巴戟天

Smooth Passage

INGREDIENTS

Sclerotium Poriae Cocos	Fu ling	茯苓
Rhizoma Atractylodis Macrocephalae	Bai zhu	白朮
Radix Paeoniae Lactiflorae	Bai shao	白芍
Radix Saussureae seu Vladimiriae	Mu xiang	木香
Rhizoma Cyperi Rotundi	Xiang fu	香附
Fructus Citri Aurantii	Zhi ke	枳殼

Cortex Phellodendri	Huang bai	黄 柏
Radix Sophorae Flavescentis	Ku shen	苦 參
Semen Nelumbins	Lian zi	蓮 子
Radix Pulsatillae	Bai tou weng	白 頭 翁
Massa Fermentata	Shen qu	神 曲

Soothe the Centre

INGREDIENTS

Rhizoma Atractylodis Macrocephalae	Bai zhu	白 朮
Radix Codonopsis Pilosulae	Dang shen	黨 參
Radix Glycyrrhizae Uralensis	Zhi gan cao	炙 甘 草
Sclerotium Poriae Cocos	Fu ling	茯 苓
Percarpium citri Reticulatae	Chen pi	陳 皮
Rhizoma Pinelliae Ternatae	Ban xia	半 夏
Fructus seu Semen Amomi	Sha ren	砂 仁
Radix Saussureae seu Vladimiriae	Mu xiang	木 香
Radix Dioscoreae Oppositae	Shan yao	山 藥
Radix Astragali	Huang qi	黄 耆
Radix Pseudostellariae Heterophyllae	Tai zi shen	太 子 參
Semen Dolichoris	Bai bian dou	白 扁 豆
Herba Angastache seu Pogostemi	Huo xiang	藿 香
Cortex Magnoliae Officinalis	Hou po	厚 樸
Folium Perillae Frutescentis	Zi su ye	紫 蘇 葉
Fructus Citri Aurantii	Zhi ke	枳 殼
Massa Fermentata	Shen qu	神 曲

Stir Field of Elixir

INGREDIENTS

Radix Linderae Strychnifoliae	Wu yao	烏 藥
Radix Angelicae Sinensis	Dang gui	當 歸
Radix Ligustici Wallichii	Chuan xiong	川 芎
Semen Persicae	Tao ren	桃 仁
Cortex Moutan Radicis	Mu dan pi	牡 丹 皮
Radix Paeoniae	Chi shao	赤 芍
Rhizoma Corydalis	Yan hu suo	延 胡 索
Radix Glycyrrhizae Uralensis	Gan cao	甘 草
Rhizoma Cyperi Rotundi	Xiang fu	香 附
Flos Carthami Tinctorii	Hong hua	紅 花
Fructus Citri Aurantii	Zhi ke	枳 殼
Pollen Typhae	Pu huang	蒲 黃
Radix Salviae Miltiorrhizae	Dan shen	丹 參
Radix Paeoniae Lactiflorae	Bai shao	白 芍

Strengthen the Root

INGREDIENTS

Radix Rehmanniae Glutinosae Conquitae	Shu di huang	熟 地 黃
Radix Dioscoreae Oppositae	Shan yao	山 藥
Fructus Corni Officinalis	Shan zhu yu	山 茱 萸
Fructus Lycii Chinensis	Gou qi zi	枸 杞 子
Cornu Cervi Parvum	Lu rong	鹿 茸
Semen Cuscutae	Tu si zi	兔 絲 子
Cortex Eucommiae Ulmoidis	Du zhong	杜 仲
Radix Angelicae Sinensis	Dang gui	當 歸
Cortex Cinnamomi Cassiae	Rou gui	肉 桂
Ramulus Cinnamomi	Gui zhi	桂 枝
Radix Glycyrrhizae Uralensis	Zhi gan cao	炙 甘 草
Radix Ginseng	Ren shen	人 參
Radix Anemarrhenae	Zhi mu	知 母

Tonify Qi and Ease the Muscles

INGREDIENTS		
Radix Astragali	Huang qi	黄 耆
Radix Ginseng	Ren shen	人 參
Rhizoma Atractylodis Macrocephalae	Bai zhu	白 朮
Radix Glycyrrhizae Uralensis	Zhi gan cao	炙 甘 草
Radix Angelicae Sinensis	Dang gui	當 歸
Percarpium citri Reticulatae	Chen pi	陳 皮
Rhizoma Cimicifugae	Sheng ma	升 麻
Radix Bupleuri	Chai hu	柴 胡
Fructus seu Semen Amomi	Sha ren	砂 仁
Herba Angastache seu Pogostemi	Huo xiang	藿 香
Semen Coicis	Yi yi ren	薏 苡 仁
Sclerotium Poriae Cocos	Fu ling	茯 苓

WOMEN'S TREASURE FORMULAE

Clear Empty Heat and Cool the Menses

INGREDIENTS		
Radix Rehmanniae	Sheng di huang	生 地 黄
Radix Paeoniae Lactiflorae	Bai shao	白 芍
Radix Dioscoreae Oppositae	Shan yao	山 藥
Radix Scutellariae Baicalensis	Huang qin	黄 芩
Cortex Phellodendri	Huang bai	黄 柏
Radix Dipsaci	Xu duan	續 斷
Herba Ecliptae Prostratae	Han lian cao	旱 蓮 草
Herba Artemisiae Annuae	Qing hao	青 蒿
Radix Sanguisorbae Officinalis	Di yu	地 榆
Radix Rubiae Cordifoliae	Qian cao gen	茜 草 根
Rhizoma Anemarrhenae Asphodeloidis	Zhi mu	知 母
Nodus Nelumbinis Nuciferae Rhizomatis	Ou jie	藕 節
Plastrum Testudinis	Gui ban	龜 板

INGREDIENTS CONTINUED FROM PAGE 260

Concha Ostreae	Mu li	牡蠣
Radix Panacis Quinquefolii	Xian he cao	仙鶴草
Cacumen Biotae Orientalis	Ce bai ye	側柏葉
Radix Glycyrrhizae Uralensis	Gan cao	甘草
Cortex Moutan Radicis	Mu dan pi	牡丹皮
Fructus Corni Officinalis	Shan zhu yu	山茱萸

Clear the Palace

INGREDIENTS

Rhizoma Pinelliae Ternatae	Ban xia	半夏
Rhizoma Atractyloidis	Cang zhu	蒼朮
Percarpium citri Reticulatae	Chen pi	陳皮
Sclerotium Poriae Cocos	Fu ling	茯苓
Rhizoma Cyperi Rotundi	Xiang fu	香附
Massa Fermentata	Shen qu	神曲
Radix Ligustici Wallichii	Chuan xiong	川芎
Semen Cuscutae	Tu si zi	菟絲子
Rhizoma Atractylodis Macrocephalae	Bai zhu	白朮
Radix Glycyrrhizae Uralensis	Gan cao	甘草
Herba Lycopi Lucidi	Ze lan	澤蘭
Fructus Liquidambaris Taiwanianae	Lu lu tong	路路通
Cortex Phellodendri	Huang bai	黄柏
Radix Cyathulae	Chuan niu xi	川牛膝
Semen Coicis	Yi yi ren	薏苡仁
Rhizoma Acori Graminei	Shi chang pu	石菖蒲

Cool the Menses

INGREDIENTS

Fructus Gardiniae Jasminoidis	Shan zhi zi	山梔子
Radix Scutellariae Baicalensis	Huang qin	黄芩
Cortex Phellodendri	Huang bai	黄柏
Radix Rehmanniae	Sheng di huang	生地黄
Cortex Moutan Radicis	Mu dan pi	牡丹皮

Radix Sanguisorbae Officinalis	Di yu	地 榆
Radix Panacis Quinquefolii	Xian he cao	仙 鶴 草
Cacumen Biotae Orientalis	Ce bai ye	側 柏 葉
Cortex Ailanthi Altissimae	Chun pi	春 皮
Gelatinum Plastri Testudinis	Gui ban jiao	龜 板 膠
Radix Paeoniae Lactiflorae	Bai shao	白 芍
Radix Rubiae Cordifoliae	Qian cao gen	茜 草 根
Pollen Typhae	Pu huang	蒲 黃
Radix Angelicae Sinensis	Dang gui	當 歸
Radix Gentianae Scabrae	Long dan cao	龍 膽 草
Radix Dipsaci	Xu duan	續 斷

Drain the Jade Valley

INGREDIENTS

Rhizoma Dioscoreae Hypogloaucae	Bei xie	萆 薢
Semen Coicis	Yi yi ren	薏 苡 仁
Cortex Phellodendri	Huang bai	黃 柏
Sclerotium Poriae Cocos	Fu ling	茯 苓
Cortex Moutan Radicis	Mu dan pi	牡 丹 皮
Rhizoma Alismatis Plantago-aquaticae	Ze xie	澤 瀉
Medulla Tetrapanacis	Tong cao	通 草
Talcum	Hua shi	滑 石
Radix Sophorae Flavescentis	Ku shen	苦 參
Fructus Meliae Toosendan	Chuan lian zi	川 楝 子
Pericarpium Arecae	Da fu pi	大 腹 皮
Fructus AlpiniaeOxyphyllae	Yi zhi ren	益 智 仁
Radix Linderae Strychnifoliae	Wu yao	烏 藥
Rhizoma Acori Graminei	Shi chang pu	石 菖 蒲
Rhizoma Atractylodis Macrocephalae	Bai zhu	白 朮
Radix Glycyrrhizae Uralensis	Gan cao	甘 草
Radix Dioscoreae Oppositae	Shan yao	山 藥
Semen Plantaginis	Che qian zi	車 前 子
Rhizoma Atractyloidis	Cang zhu	蒼 朮
Radix Cyathulae	Chuan niu xi	川 牛 膝

Drain Redness

INGREDIENTS

Cortex Moutan Radicis	Mu dan pi	牡 丹 皮
Radix Rehmanniae	Sheng di huang	生 地 黃
Cortex Phellodendri	Huang bai	黃 柏
Radix Angelicae Sinensis	Dang gui	當 歸
Radix Paeoniae Lactiflorae	Bai shao	白 芍
Radix Paeoniae	Chi shao	赤 芍
Radix Ligustici Wallichii	Chuan xiong	川 芎
Flos Carthami Tinctorii	Hong hua	紅 花
Semen Persicae	Tao ren	桃 仁
Rhizoma Corydalis	Yan hu suo	延 胡 索
Herba Leonuri Heterophylli	Yi mu cao	益 母 草
Semen Plantaginis	Che qian zi	車 前 子
Radix Gentianae Scabrae	Long dan cao	龍 膽 草

Female Treasure

INGREDIENTS

Radix Rehmanniae	Sheng di huang	生 地 黃
Tuber Asparagi Cochinchinensis	Tian men dong	天 門 冬
Radix Paeoniae Lactiflorae	Bai shao	白 芍
Frutus Ligustri Lucidi	Nu zhen zi	女 貞 子
Flos Chrysanthemi Morifolii	Ju hua	菊 花
Radix Scutellariae Baicalensis	Huang qin	黃 芩
Semen Zizyphi Spinosae	Suan zao ren	酸 棗 仁
Os Draconis	Long gu	龍 骨
Fructus Lycii Chinensis	Gou qi zi	枸 杞 子
Fructus Corni Officinalis	Shan zhu yu	山 茱 萸
Radix Dioscoreae Oppositae	Shan yao	山 藥
Rhizoma Alismatis Plantago-aquaticae	Ze xie	澤 瀉
Cortex Moutan Radicis	Mu dan pi	牡 丹 皮
Sclerotium Poriae Cocos	Fu ling	茯 苓
Plastrum Testudinis	Gui ban	龜 板
Concha Ostreae	Mu li	牡 蠣

Radix Gentianae Macrophyllae	Qin jiao	秦 艽
Cortex Lycii Radicis	Di gu pi	地 骨 皮
Fructus Oryzae	Gu ya	谷 芽

Growing Jade

INGREDIENTS

Radix Angelicae Sinensis	Dang gui	當 歸
Radix Paeoniae Lactiflorae	Bai shao	白 芍
Radix Rehmanniae Glutinosae Conquitae	Shu di huang	熟 地 黄
Fructus Corni Officinalis	Shan zhu yu	山 茱 萸
Frutus Ligustri Lucidi	Nu zhen zi	女 貞 子
Herba Ecliptae Prostratae	Han lian cao	旱 蓮 草
Radix Rehmanniae	Sheng di huang	生 地 黄
Fructus Lycii Chinensis	Gou qi zi	枸 杞 子
Herba Leonuri Heterophylli	Yi mu cao	益 母 草
Radix Dioscoreae Oppositae	Shan yao	山 藥
Radix Morindae Officinalis	Ba ji tian	巴 戟 天
Plastrum Testudinis	Gui ban	龜 板
Semen Cuscutae	Tu si zi	兔 絲 子
Rhizoma Polygonati	Huang jing	黄 精
Sclerotium Poriae Cocos	Fu ling	茯 苓

Heavenly Empress

INGREDIENTS

Radix Rehmanniae	Sheng di huang	生 地 黄
Radix Scorphulariae Ning poensis	Xuan shen	玄 參
Tuber Ophiopogonis Japonici	Mai men dong	麥 門 冬
Tuber Asparagi Cochinchinensis	Tian men dong	天 門 冬
Gelatinum Plastri Testudinis	Gui ban jiao	龜 板 膠
Radix Ginseng	Ren shen	人 參
Sclerotium Poriae Cocos	Fu ling	茯 苓
Frutus Schisandrae Chinensis	Wu wei zi	五 味 子
Radix Angelicae Sinensis	Dang gui	當 歸

Radix Salviae Miltiorrhizae	Dan shen	丹 參
Semen Biotae Orientalis	Bai zhi ren	柏 智 仁
Semen Zizyphi Spinosae	Suan zao ren	酸 棗 仁
Radix Polygale Tenuifoliae Recens	Yuan zhi	遠 志
Radix Platycodi Grandiflori	Jie geng	桔 梗
Radix Gentianae Macrophyllae	Qin jiao	秦 艽
Herba Artemisiae Annuae	Qing hao	青 蒿
Cortex Lycii Radicis	Di gu pi	地 骨 皮
Cortex Moutan Radicis	Mu dan pi	牡 丹 皮
Concha Ostreae	Mu li	牡 蠣
Fructus Lycii Chinensis	Gou qi zi	枸 杞 子

Invigorate Blood and Stem the Flow

INGREDIENTS

Radix Angelicae Sinensis	Dang gui	當 歸
Radix Ligustici Wallichii	Chuan xiong	川 芎
Radix Rehmanniae	Sheng di huang	生 地 黃
Radix Paeoniae Lactiflorae	Bai shao	白 芍
Semen Persicae	Tao ren	桃 仁
Flos Carthami Tinctorii	Hong hua	紅 花
Pollen Typhae	Pu huang	蒲 黃
Radix Rubiae Cordifoliae	Qian cao gen	茜 草 根
Radix Pseudoginseng	San qi	三 七
Radix Panacis Quinquefolii	Xian he cao	仙 鶴 草
Radix Salviae Miltiorrhizae	Dan shen	丹 參
Rhizoma Cyperi Rotundi	Xiang fu	香 附
Radix Paeoniae	Chi shao	赤 芍
Cortex Moutan Radicis	Mu dan pi	牡 丹 皮
Fructus Corni Officinalis	Shan zhu yu	山 茱 萸

Nourish Yin and Restrain the Flow

INGREDIENTS

Radix Rehmanniae	Sheng di huang	生 地 黄
Radix Dioscoreae Oppositae	Shan yao	山 藥
Fructus Corni Officinalis	Shan zhu yu	山 茱 萸
Fructus Lycii Chinensis	Gou qi zi	枸 杞 子
Semen Cuscutae	Tu si zi	兎 絲 子
Cornu Cervi Degelatinatium	Lu jiao jiao	鹿 角 膠
Gelatinum Plastri Testudinis	Gui ban jiao	龜 板 膠
Frutus Ligustri Lucidi	Nu zhen zi	女 貞 子
Radix Anemarrhenae	Zhi mu	知 母
Radix Paeoniae Lactiflorae	Bai shao	白 芍
Herba Ecliptae Prostratae	Han lian cao	旱 蓮 草
Gelatinum Asini	E jiao	阿 膠
Radix Panacis Quinquefolii	Xian he cao	仙 鶴 草
Cacumen Biotae Orientalis	Ce bai ye	側 柏 葉
Concha Ostreae	Mu li	牡 蠣
Sclerotium Poriae Cocos	Fu ling	茯 苓
Fructus Oryzae	Gu ya	谷 芽

Penetrating Vessel

INGREDIENTS

Plastri Testudinis	Gui ban	龜 板
Radix Rehmanniae Glutinosae Conquitae	Shu di huang	熟 地 黄
Radix Paeoniae Lactiflorae	Bai shao	白 芍
Radix Angelicae Sinensis	Dang gui	當 歸
Semen Cuscutae	Tu si zi	兎 絲 子
Fructus foeniculi Vulgaris	Xiao hui xiang	小 茴 香
Rhizoma Corydalis	Yan hu suo	延 胡 索
Rhizoma Cyperi Rotundi	Xiang fu	香 附
Fructus Meliae Toosendan	Chuan lian zi	川 楝 子
Fructus Leonturi	Chong wei zi	茺 蔚 子
Pericarpium Citri Reticulatae Viride	Qing pi	青 皮
Cortex Albizziae Julibrissin	He huan pi	合 歡 皮

INGREDIENTS CONTINUED FROM PAGE 266

Rhizoma Pinelliae Ternatae	Ban xia	半 夏
Radix Salviae Miltiorrhizae	Dan shen	丹 參
Cortex Magnoliae Officinalis	Hou po	厚 樸
Radix Asteris Tatarici	Zi wan	紫 苑
Folium Perillae Frutescentis	Zi su ye	紫 蘇 葉
Radix Glycyrrhizae Uralensis	Gan cao	甘 草

Planting Seeds

INGREDIENTS

Semen Cuscutae	Tu si zi	兔 絲 子
Radix Dipsaci	Xu duan	續 斷
Radix Morindae Officinalis	Ba ji tian	巴 戟 天
Cortex Eucommiae Ulmoidis	Du zhong	杜 仲
Cornu Cervi Degelatinatium	Lu jiao shuang	鹿 角 霜
Radix Angelicae Sinensis	Dang gui	當 歸
Radix Rehmanniae Glutinosae Conquitae	Shu di huang	熟 地 黃
Fructus Lycii Chinensis	Gou qi zi	枸 杞 子
Gelatinum Asini	E jiao	阿 膠
Radix Ginseng	Ren shen	人 參
Rhizoma Atractylodis Macrocephalae	Bai zhu	白 朮
Fructus Zizyphi Jujubae	Da zao	大 棗
Fructus seu Semen Amomi	Sha ren	砂 仁
Rhizoma Cimicifugae	Sheng ma	升 麻
Radix Dioscoreae Oppositae	Shan yao	山 藥
Gelatinum Plastri Testudinis	Gui ban jiao	龜 板 膠
Radix Scutellariae Baicalensis	Huang qin	黃 芩

Precious Sea

INGREDIENTS

Radix Angelicae Sinensis	Dang gui	當 歸
Radix Rehmanniae Glutinosae Conquitae	Shu di huang	熟 地 黄
Radix Paeoniae Lactiflorae	Bai shao	白 芍
Radix Ligustici Wallichii	Chuan xiong	川 芎
Radix Codonopsis Pilosulae	Dang shen	黨 參
Rhizoma Atractylodis Macrocephalae	Bai zhu	白 朮
Radix Astragali	Huang qi	黄 耆
Radix Ginseng	Ren shen	人 參
Sclerotium Poriae Cocos	Fu ling	茯 苓
Radix Glycyrrhizae Uralensis	Zhi gan cao	炙 甘 草
Herba Leonuri Heterophylli	Yi mu cao	益 母 草
Rhizoma Cyperi Rotundi	Xiang fu	香 附
Radix Polygoni Multiflori	Shou wu	首 烏
Fructus Lycii Chinensis	Gou qi zi	枸 杞 子
Semen Cuscutae	Tu si zi	兎 絲 子
Rhizoma Polygonati	Huang jing	黄 精
Semen Biotae Orientalis	Bai zi ren	柏 子 仁

Restrain the Flow

INGREDIENTS

Radix Astragali	Huang qi	黄 耆
Radix Ginseng	Ren shen	人 參
Rhizoma Atractylodis Macrocephalae	Bai zhu	白 朮
Radix Rehmanniae Glutinosae Conquitae	Shu di huang	熟 地 黄
Radix Angelicae Sinensis	Dang gui	當 歸
Radix Panacis Quinquefolii	Xian he cao	仙 鶴 草
Cacumen Biotae Orientalis	Ce bai ye	側 柏 葉
Herba seu Flos Schizonepetae Tenuifoliae	Jing jie	荆 芥
Radix Dipsaci	Xu duan	續 斷
Semen Cuscutae	Tu si zi	兎 絲 子
Rhizoma Cimicifugae	Sheng ma	升 麻
Radix Glycyrrhizae Uralensis	Gan cao	甘 草
Fructus Corni Officinalis	Shan zhu yu	山 茱 萸

Stir Field of Elixir

INGREDIENTS

Radix Linderae Strychnifoliae	Wu yao	烏 藥
Radix Angelicae Sinensis	Dang gui	當 歸
Radix Ligustici Wallichii	Chuan xiong	川 芎
Semen Persicae	Tao ren	桃 仁
Cortex Moutan Radicis	Mu dan pi	牡 丹 皮
Radix Paeoniae	Chi shao	赤 芍
Rhizoma Corydalis	Yan hu suo	延 胡 索
Radix Glycyrrhizae Uralensis	Gan cao	甘 草
Rhizoma Cyperi Rotundi	Xiang fu	香 附
Flos Carthami Tinctorii	Hong hua	紅 花
Fructus Citri Aurantii	Zhi ke	枳 殼
Pollen Typhae	Pu huang	蒲 黃
Radix Salviae Miltiorrhizae	Dan shen	丹 參
Radix Paeoniae Lactiflorae	Bai shao	白 芍

Unicorn Pearl

INGREDIENTS

Radix Ginseng	Ren shen	人 參
Rhizoma Atractylodis Macrocephalae	Bai zhu	白 朮
Radix Paeoniae Lactiflorae	Bai shao	白 芍
Radix Glycyrrhizae Uralensis	Zhi gan cao	炙 甘 草
Radix Angelicae Sinensis	Dang gui	當 歸
Radix Rehmanniae Glutinosae Conquitae	Shu di huang	熟 地 黃
Semen Cuscutae	Tu si zi	兎 絲 子
Cortex Eucommiae Ulmoidis	Du zhong	杜 仲
Radix Dipsaci	Xu duan	續 斷
Cornu Cervi Degelatinatium	Lu jiao jiao	鹿 角 膠

Warm the Mansion

INGREDIENTS

Ramulus Cinnamomi	Gui zhi	桂 枝
Folium Artemisiae Argyi	Ai ye	艾 葉
Fructus Evodiae	Wu zhu yu	吳 茱 萸
Cortex Cinnamomi Cassiae	Rou gui	肉 桂
Rhizoma Cyperi Rotundi	Xiang fu	香 附
Radix Linderae Strychnifoliae	Wu yao	烏 藥
Radix Angelicae Sinensis	Dang gui	當 歸
Radix Ligustici Wallichii	Chuan xiong	川 芎
Radix Paeoniae Lactiflorae	Bai shao	白 芍
Radix Dipsaci	Xu duan	續 斷
Semen Cuscutae	Tu si zi	菟 絲 子
Herba Epimedii	Yin yang huo	淫 羊 藿
Semen Citri Reticulatae	Ju he	桔 核
Semen Litchi Chinensis	Li zhi he	荔 枝 核
Fructus foeniculi Vulgaris	Xiao hui xiang	小 茴 香
Cortex Moutan Radicis	Mu dan pi	牡 丹 皮

Warm the Menses

INGREDIENTS

Fructus Evodiae	Wu zhu yu	吳 茱 萸
Ramulus Cinnamomi	Gui zhi	桂 枝
Cortex Cinnamomi Cassiae	Rou gui	肉 桂
Radix Angelicae Sinensis	Dang gui	當 歸
Radix Ligustici Wallichii	Chuan xiong	川 芎
Radix Paeoniae Lactiflorae	Bai shao	白 芍
Radix Codonopsis Pilosulae	Dang shen	黨 參
Tuber Ophiopogonis Japonici	Mai men dong	麥 門 冬
Radix Rehmanniae Glutinosae Conquitae	Shu di huang	熟 地 黃
Cortex Moutan Radicis	Mu dan pi	牡 丹 皮
Rhizoma Pinelliae Ternatae	Ban xia	半 夏
Radix Glycyrrhizae Uralensis	Zhi gan cao	炙 甘 草
Rhizoma Corydalis	Yan hu suo	延 胡 索
Radix Linderae Strychnifoliae	Wu yao	烏 藥
Herba Leonuri Heterophylli	Yi mu cao	益 母 草
Cortex Eucommiae Ulmoidis	Du zhong	杜 仲

Symptom Reference Index

Patent Medicine Index

Glossary of Chinese Medical Terms

Chong mai "Penetrating Vessel"; one of the eight extraordinary or "irregular" meridians; involved in reproduction and menstruation.

Dai mai "Girdle Vessel"; one of the eight extra or irregular meridians; important in regulating the upward and downward flow of *qi* in the body.

Eight extraordinary meridians Eight extraordinary meridians or "vessels," so named because they are not interconnected and serve as reservoirs that act as receptacles in excess conditions and sources in deficient conditions; these meridians are accessed through points on the twelve regular meridians.

Fu organ "Hollow" organs, classified as *yang* organs; involved in the transport of nutrients and waste through and out of the body. Includes large intestine, small intestine, stomach, gallbladder, urinary bladder, and *san jiao*. (*See* Zang organs.)

Jiao "Burner" or "warmer." Any of three specific regions (collectively the *san*, or three, *jiao*) of the thorax and its organs: the upper *jiao* is the region above the diaphragm and includes the heart and lungs; the middle *jiao* is the region from the diaphragm to the navel and includes the spleen and stomach; the lower *jiao* is the region from the navel to the upper border of the pubic bone and includes the liver and kidneys.

Jueyin "Extreme" or "terminal" *yin*. Includes two of the six *yin* meridians: the liver and pericardium.

Meridian From the Chinese term *jing* (to go through) *luo* (something that connects, like a network). A meridian is a pathway through which *qi* and blood pass that comprises part of a circulatory network throughout the body.

Qi A concept that might imperfectly be considered "vital energy" or "vital substance." In broader terms, *qi* is the fundamental substance that constitutes the universe and whose actions control all phenomena; in terms of Traditional Chinese Medicine, *qi* is the material basis for and governs all of the functions of the human body. Note: There is no Western equivalent to the term *qi*, partly because the Chinese conceive of *qi* more in terms of what it *does* than what it *is*.

Qi hua Refers to the functions of certain organs, such as the urinary bladder.

Ren mai "Conception vessel." One of the eight extraordinary meridians or vessels; involved in reproduction and menstruation.

San jiao "Three burners" or "Triple warmer." The region of the thorax from the clavicle to the upper border of the pubic bone; a *yang* organ with no Western counterpart, thought to be integral to the metabolism of fluids in the body. (*See* jiao.)

Sea of Blood One of the names of the *Chong mai*. (*See* Chong mai.)

Shaoyang "Lesser yang." Includes two of the six yang meridians: the gallbladder and *san jiao*.

Shen "Consciousness" or "spirit." Involves mental activities such as the capacity to think and desire.

Shi "Excess" or "full." Refers to a condition of imbalance, ultimately of the archetypes of *yin* and *yang*, within the human body. (*See* xu.)

Wei qi "Defensive" *qi*; outermost layer of bodily *qi* that protects from external pathogenic invasions.

Xu "Deficient" or "empty." Refers to a condition of imbalance, ultimately of the archetypes of *yin* and *yang*, within the human body. (*See* shi.)

Yin and yang A pair of archetypal principles that exist in constant opposition to and dependence on each other; the pair as a whole compromise reality itself, and their tension is reflected in the dynamic nature of the universe. The original meanings of the terms were the sunny part of a hill (*yang*) and the shaded, or back, part of a hill (*yin*). In the human body, *yang* represents the heating, energetic, functional aspects, while *yin* represents the cooling, fluid, material aspects.

Ying qi "Nutrient" *qi*; type of *qi* derived from the digestive organs that helps in the production and circulation of blood.

Zang organs "Solid" organs, classified as yin organs. Involved in the production and storage of *qi*, blood, and body fluids. Includes heart, lungs, pericardium, spleen, liver, and kidney.

List of Suppliers

CHINA HERB COMPANY
6333 Wayne Avenue
Philadelphia, PA 19144
Tel: 1-800-221-432
Fax: (215) 849-3338

CHINESE MODULAR SOLUTIONS
Tel: (415) 285-0931

EAST TAO HERB PHARMACY
2801 Rodeo Road #F
Santa Fe, NM 87505
Tel: (505) 438-7178
Fax: (505) 438-1056

GOLDEN FLOWER CHINESE HERBS
P.O. Box 781
Placitas, NM 87043
Tel: 1-800-729-8509

HEALTH CONCERNS
8001 Capwell Drive
Oakland, CA 94621
Tel: 1-800-233-9355
Fax: (510) 639-9140

JADE PHARMACY
East Earth Herb, Inc.
P.O. Box 2802
Eugene, OR 97402
Tel: 1-800-827-4372

K'AN HERBALS
6001 Butler Lane
Scotts Valley, CA 95066
Tel: (408) 438-9450
Fax: (408) 438-9457

LONG LIFE HERBAL PHARMACY
6329 15th Avenue NE
Seattle, WA 98115
Tel: 1-800-829-2126 or (206) 522-0910
Fax: (209) 525-4379

METAGENICS, INC.
971 Calle Negocio
San Clemente, CA 92673
Tel: 1-800-692-9400

PACIFIC BIOLOGIC
P.O. Box 520
Clayton, CA 94517-0520
Tel: 1-800-829-2126
Fax: (510) 673-2966

PRO BOTANIXX
9200 Jeronimo Road
Irvine, CA 92618
Tel: 1-800-909-4372
Fax: (714) 457-6038

THE THREE TREASURES/ WOMEN'S TREASURES
East West Herb, Ltd.
6400 Hollis Street,
Suite 10
Emeryville, CA 94608
Tel: 1-800-575-8526